Ageing

By the same author

IN SEARCH OF NIRVANA: A NEW PERSPECTIVE ON
ALCOHOL AND DRUG DEPENDENCY

Dr Ghadirian's book, which is based on strong spiritual beliefs, deals with issues concerning the very fabric of our lives: Why do we age? What comes after death? All readers will learn something from this book. Health professionals who work with Alzheimer's patients will find some refreshing suggestions.

A healthy physical, intellectual and spiritual life style may well have a positive influence on the ageing process. This book enables us to take a step towards such a life style.

Serge Gauthier, MD, FRCP(C)
Director, McGill Centre for Studies in Ageing
Professor of Neurology and Neurosurgery,
McGill University

Ageing

Challenges and Opportunities

by

A-M. Ghadirian

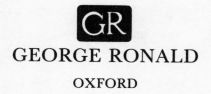

GEORGE RONALD

OXFORD

GEORGE RONALD, Publisher
46 High Street, Kidlington, Oxford OX5 2DN

British Library Cataloguing in Publication Data

Ghadirian, A-M.
    Ageing: challenges and opportunities
    I. Title
    305.26

ISBN 0–85398–329–1

Contents

Preface   ix
Introduction   1
  Ageing: An Historical Perspective   1
  Ageing: Definition and Types   4
  Predictors of Psychosocial Health in Later Life   7
  Middle Age: A Period of Stabilization   8
  Challenges of Old Age   10
  Creativity in Old Age   10

1 Our Ageing Society: Some Statistics and
  Reflections   12
  'Young' and 'Old' as Symbols   12
  The Rise of an Ageing Population   14
  Factors Contributing to an 'Ageing Society'   18
  Contemporary Ageing Society: A Demographic View   18
  Myths and Misconceptions about Ageing   19

2 The Psychobiological Clock   22
  Environment and the Aged   25
  Tranquillity in Old Age   26

3 Ageing and Creativity   28
  The Value of the Elderly in Society   38

4 The Challenges of Old Age   41

Attitudes towards the Elderly   42
Physical and Psychological Challenges of Old Age   42
Some Defence Mechanisms   45
Spiritual Responses to Old Age   49
Some Other Psychological Challenges of Old Age   50

5 Coping with Stress   57
The Meaning of Stress   58
Individual Responses to Stress   59
Societal Attitudes towards Stress   63
Stress and Personality   65
Biological Responses to Stress   65
How to Cope with Stress   66
The Spiritual Dimension   74

6 Alzheimer's Disease: An Eclipse before Sunset   76
Biological Dimensions   77
Psychosocial Dimensions   78
Spiritual Dimensions   80
Intelligence and Understanding   83
Mental Illness and the Soul   84
Caring Attitude   84
Family Observations of Alzheimer Patients   85
Caring for Patients with Alzheimer's Disease:
    A Family Challenge   90
Misconceptions about Alzheimer Patients   94
The Responsibility of the Care-Givers   95
Stress in Caring for Alzheimer Patients   97
Caring for Care-Givers   98
The Role of Society   99
Some Suggestions for Caring   102

7 Ageing: A Spiritual Perspective   110

CONTENTS vii

The Evolution of the Soul 110
The Sensory and Spiritual Powers 112
The Decline of the Physical Senses 113
Intellectual Powers and Ageing 113
Spiritual Development Knows No Age 114
Spiritual Health 115
Preparation for the Next World 116
Needs of the Next World 117
The Rewards of Life in this World and the Next 118

References 120

This book is a tribute to all
travellers on the journey of life

Preface

Ageing is not an isolated phenomenon which occurs 'out there'. It is very much part of our personal day-to-day experience. It is a process through which we grow and mature and contribute to our family and to society.

Ageing is a universal phenomenon, yet we know very little about it. Until recently, traditional education focused primarily on early development and growth, and not much attention was given to the process of ageing and old age itself.

With advances in science and medicine, life expectancy has increased; thus the number of elderly people in the population is on the rise. More and more people are able to celebrate their seventieth, eightieth, ninetieth and even one hundredth birthdays. It is estimated that, worldwide, one in every five males and almost two in every five females can expect to live to the age of 85.

Governments, educators and health professionals are beginning to realize the implications of this growth in the number of aged people in the population. In the United States alone there are more than 25 million people over the age of 65. Of these, more than 6.2 million are aged 80 or over, putting the United States at the top of the list of nine countries which have more than a million octogenarians. By the year 2025, the United States, China, the Soviet Union, India, Japan, Germany, France, England and Italy will be joined by nine other countries having more than a million people aged 80 or

over. China is expected to emerge as the country with the
largest octogenarian population (estimated to be 26.4 million)
followed by India (16.4 million) and the United States (14.3
million). The most rapid growth in the aged population has
occurred in Japan where the number of people aged 65 and
over has doubled in the past 20 years.

With this unprecedented increase in the number of elderly
people, societies are facing challenges never before encountered. For example, as rising numbers of older people choose
to stay in their own homes, no one knows how many care-
givers will be available to look after them, how the health
system will be able to provide adequate care for them, or how
the life style of younger family members who live with their
elderly relatives will be affected. We do know that many
elderly people will require specialized medical attention and
that preventative medicine and health education will be
important aspects of their care.

Faced with this development, society needs to re-examine
its attitude towards and treatment of its ageing population. It
is time to cast away our prejudices towards ageing and old age
and come to terms with the reality of this final and most
enriching period of the human journey on this plane of
existence. We need to rethink the pattern and organization of
our communities so that the newly-emerging society will be
one in which the rights and welfare of the elderly are
recognized and protected.

It has only been in recent years that the mystery of ageing
and old age has begun to unfold. People have the right to be
educated about the process and prospects of ageing and about
the art of ageing with dignity. Historically, most people did
not live long enough to experience the vicissitudes of old age
as we know them. Today people are asking, 'How do we age?
What is the efect of ageing on our muscles and our minds?
How do we cope with stress in old age? How do we face losses

in later life? What can we do about loneliness and isolation? Where shall we turn if poverty strikes or violence breaks out? How can we manage if memory fails or dementia overtakes us?'

In addition to these concerns, people also hold cherished hopes and dreams – dreams of seeing grandchildren grow up and the new generation prosper. Many have a renewed interest in serving, creating and discovering the mystery of life.

Ageing is neither free from pain nor free from joy. We need to learn about it as we do about any aspect of human development. We have been taught how to climb the high mountain of life but once at the top we do not know how to come down, as eventually we must, gracefully.

One of the most neglected areas of ageing is its spiritual dimension. The spiritual reality of ageing and old age is central to our recognition of the meaning and purpose of life. This book is concerned not only with the psychosocial aspects of ageing but also with its spiritual meaning.

My interest in the life of elderly people developed through my personal experience with those who are dear to me as well as through my professional involvement with the elderly. Whether by their joy or their sorrow, their humour or their wisdom, the elderly individuals whom I have known have all inspired me. This book is a tribute to them.

The preparation of this book was a long process which became a journey of my own into the mystery of ageing. Each chapter confronted me with a new realization and brought forth a new reflection upon the reality of our transitory life in this world. This book is not intended to be an exhaustive work on issues relating to geriatric problems and their treatment; rather it is my hope to explore new frontiers in understanding the challenges and opportunites of old age.

I would like to express my sincere gratitude to all those who assisted me in my task. To name a few, I am grateful to Dr Martin Cole, Dr Jacqueline McClaran, Dr Serge Gauthier and Dr May Ballerio who read the manuscript and inspired me with their advice and encouragement. I am also deeply grateful to Phoebe Ann Lemmon and Elizabeth Rochester for providing material from their own experience and to Louise Polland for editorial corrections. In particular I am indebted to Dr Wendi Momen for her valuable suggestions and final editing of the manuscript. I am profoundly grateful to my wife, Marilyn, for her loving support and tireless assistance in the preparation of this book. I also thank our sons Sina and Nayyer for their patience and understanding which allowed me to bring this project to its completion.

A-M. Ghadirian
Mount Royal, Quebec
April 1991

Introduction

Elderly people will constitute a very large proportion of the world's population by the year 2000. This change in the composition of the population will require a major change in our attitudes and activities, something for which we have only a very few years to prepare. As the number of elderly people grows, concern for their well-being is expressed by greater numbers of family members and other care-givers. The elderly themselves share such concerns. However, while acknowledging the many challenges which an ageing population presents to society, we must also recognize that this last stage of human development offers many opportunities for personal growth and for the growth of the family and community.

Ageing: An Historical Perspective

Among the early literate societies of the world, the ancient Hebrew civilization is one of the earliest for which there are written records with regard to the aged. The ancient Hebrews also established one of the first societies in which a long life was considered to be a blessing and not a burden.[1] It has been noted that in the years between 1300 BC and 100 AD the Hebrews were a nomadic desert tribe which was basically one large extended family consisting of wives and children as well as slaves, servants and others who joined this tribe.

They were ruled by the eldest man, the patriarch of the family, who was the religious leader, judge and teacher. He controlled all aspects of political, religious, economic and social life and was identified by his long grey beard – a sign of wisdom, experience and authority. In this relatively stable yet nomadic culture, ageing, at least for men, represented increasing wisdom, respect and power.[2]

However not all ancient societies respected the elderly. Indeed, in some pre-literate societies, the aged were abandoned or killed because they were perceived as a burden to society. This practice existed particularly among the nomads.

Of special interest in more recent times are the Abkhasians of the Georgian Republic of the Soviet Union. Society in this population is organized around collective farms located in rural villages of the Caucasus Mountains in the southern part of the USSR. The population of this region is noted for its longevity and vitality.[3] According to some estimates, about 2.6% of the population of this area is over 90 years old, compared to only 0.1% of the population throughout the rest of the USSR.

In the Abkhasian society the elderly are highly valued and as they grow old their prestige and importance increases. Indeed, people of this region long to appear older than their actual age so as to be given higher status. Barry McPherson noted that,

The Abkhasians work at their own pace from childhood to death and are never fully retired. Throughout, there is stability in lifestyle with an emphasis on the attitude that work is essential for everyone, regardless of age. These people appear physically younger than their years and they have the culturally induced expectation and the hope that they will live long lives.

Although an explanation for this longevity is lacking,

heredity, combined with various sociocultural factors seems to account for the extended life. Longevity in this sub-culture may be influenced by many factors: a system of folk medicine; a low-calorie, low-cholesterol diet of vegetables and milk, lack of competition among workers; and a strong bond with a large extended family, including non-relatives who have the same surname. All of these combine to provide a serene, secure, and healthy life style.[4]

However, this traditional life style and cultural pattern has been changing due to a new attitude of the young generation towards nutrition. Moreover, the Soviet government's decision to introduce competition into the collective system has also contributed to the change.

In the West, the industrial revolution changed people's attitudes towards themselves and towards the elderly. In the pre-industrial era there were two types of societies. One type consisted of the primitive and hunting-and-gathering societies. The oldest member of the community was a person who was very knowledgeable in rituals and survival skills. In some of these societies authority was linked to age and consequently many of the elderly people occupied important social, religious and political positions. In other societies the elderly occupied other important roles such as 'advisory', 'contributory', 'control', and 'residual' aspects of community functioning. These were considered prestige-generating components of the life of the elderly. In most of the pre-industrial societies the aged had meaningful roles so long as they were physically and mentally fit to contribute to the welfare of the family and community. They retained considerable influence and power in the social and political fabric of the society.

However, not all pre-industrial societies treated the elderly with dignity. Indeed, in some societies they were discriminated against and were forced to die. The relatives would contribute to this predicament as they considered the elderly to be a burden to the community. With the advancement of the industrial revolution, technological progress brought considerable comfort and prosperity. However, these positive changes did not necessarily bring peace and prosperity for the aged population. In societies where technological advancement brought dehumanization of human values, the elderly were deemed a burden. They were denied their rights and dignity as they were no longer productive. In countries where the extended family was preserved, the elderly had a better chance of being cared for and looked after. The universal medicare system established in some societies has helped elderly people to receive better care and treatment. In some countries mandatory retirement has been removed and replaced with a more flexible attitude, allowing elderly people to work longer.

Ageing: Definition and Types

The word 'ageing' comes from the Latin *aetas* meaning 'age' or 'lifetime'.[5] To age is to grow old, to ripen or to become mature over a period of time. 'Gerontology', used for the first time in 1903 by Metchnikoff of the Pasteur Institute in Paris, stems from the Greek word for old man (*geron*) and *logos* (knowledge) and refers to the science devoted to the study of ageing. Six years later, in New York, Ignatius Leo Nascher coined the word 'geriatrics' to speak about the clinical aspects of the ageing process.[6] There is also a difference between the terms 'ageing' and 'senescence' in that the former refers to the process of growing old or adding on years regardless of one's age, whereas the latter refers to being old or becoming older once one is already old.

McPherson divides ageing into four types as follows:[7]

Chronological ageing This is a type of ageing which is characterized by the passage of calendar time. Its passage influences lifestyle and stages of human development. For example, the age at which a person begins school, joins Scouts, or is allowed to apply for a licence to drive a car or to vote in civic elections is decided by chronological age. This is the age society uses to determine when it is legal for its members to engage in certain human activities.

Biological ageing This type of ageing refers to internal and external changes involving bodily function and structure. Human longevity and behaviour are closely related to this phenomenon. For example, as a result of slowness in psycho-motor activities, it takes longer to respond or to react on reflex. Biological changes also include greying of hair, increased subcutaneous fat, decreased functional activity of kidneys and decline of skin and vascular elasticity. Although susceptibility to diseases increases with ageing, the latter is not by itself an illness. Biological ageing will have psychological consequences depending on the personality profile of the individual. For example, in women, menopause and its associated hormonal alterations and the cessation of repro-ductivity may cause behavioural changes. Such a change in behaviour largely depends on a woman's sense of fulfilment or lack of it during the preceding child-bearing years. Thus two women of the same age may have two entirely different perceptions of ageing depending on their life styles and their characters in their earlier years.

Genetics and environment, also referred to as 'nature and nurture' factors, are involved in this process. One outcome is senescence and old age. Human senses and organs are affected by the interaction of external and internal functions. For example, the advancement of biological ageing may be associated with changes in the colour or growth of hair, the texture of skin, the strength of eyesight, the function of internal organs, and the stature and posture of an individual. The intensity of such changes may determine the number of years that a person is expected to survive.

Psychological ageing This is a type of ageing which is associated with changes in personality, memory, motivation and creativity as well as the ability to develop skills and to learn. As in biological ageing, the interaction between the internal and external factors constitutes the hallmark of psychological ageing. For example, the decline of hearing, vision and attention span may lead to discontinuation of certain activities, such as reading or sports and consequently may alter the life style of the individual. Likewise, the loss of a loved one such as a spouse (an external factor) may cause behavioural changes such as depression (internal process).

Social ageing Social ageing refers to the influence of society on the development of the individual and his social status. Ageing in this context is a social process which varies from culture to culture.

Some authors divide ageing into two types, primary and secondary.[8] Primary ageing is caused by genetic and biological factors which are time dependent. Secondary ageing is a result of diseases and other psychobiological impairments.[9] Two categories of theories about ageing have been generated from them: one category considers ageing to be genetically programmed while the other views it in terms of damage to the body.

The 'programmed' theories are based on the notion that ageing is programmed at birth, just as is puberty, and that a

person's life span is determined by heredity.[10] Supporting
evidence for the genetic theory of ageing includes the
similarities found in the life span of identical twins as well as
the fact that children of long-lived parents tend to live longer
than those who come from families which have a shorter life
span. Moreover, certain conditions such as Down's syndrome
are known to shorten life span.[11]

On the other hand, 'damage' theories maintain that
individuals throughout their lives accumulate wear-and-tear
which limits the natural ability of the biological system to
maintain and repair itself.[12] Damage can be on many levels,
such as that which may occur to the genetic element or DNA
(deoxyribonucleic acid, related to RNA, ribonucleic acid,
mentioned elsewhere in this book).

These contrasting hypotheses together with other current
theories indicate that a unified and universally acceptable
theory of normal ageing is lacking at present. This may be due
to the fact that our knowledge of medicine is still in a stage of
infancy. On the other hand, there have been impressive
discoveries and important progress in the field of gerontology
in this century. Today, the science of ageing is one of the most
rapidly expanding fields of health science in schools of
medicine.

Predictors of Psychosocial Health in Later Life

Researchers at Harvard University studied the psychosocial
health and adjustment of 173 male students who entered that
university in the 1940s. These students, initially college
sophomores, were followed for 45 years from the age of 18 to
65 or until the time of their death. They were regularly
examined and their state of health was recorded. The
researchers[13] examined certain biological and psychosocial

predictors gathered from this population before age 50. Some of the important predictive factors of good or poor health in later life were related to whether or not the man's relationship with his parents as a child were conducive to trust, autonomy and initiative. Closeness with siblings also played an important role in the psychosocial outcome of later age.[14] Those who used tranquillizers before the age of 50 were more likely to have an unhealthy mental and physical life at 65.[15]

According to this study, five important factors which probably play an important role in adjustment to later life were: 1. long-lived ancestors (important factor in physical health only); 2. sustained familial relationships (including previous closeness to parents and also prior closeness to siblings); 3. maturity of human defences; 4. absence of alcoholism; and 5. absence of depression at earlier ages.[16]

Middle Age: A Period of Stabilization

In order to understand the place of old age in our development over a lifetime, let us look first at the stage of life that precedes it – middle age. There is no clear consensus about the definition or length of middle age even though it is very much in people's minds. Researchers and authors differ in their views on this matter. Many agree that the period of middle age begins at age 45 and ends at 65. However, it has also been suggested that middle age begins as early as 35 years and ends as late as 70. According to some researchers, middle age may have nothing to do with the years of life; rather, it is related to landmarks in life, that is to say, important events characteristic of this period of life. The landmarks may be important events in one's life, such as menopause, reaching the peak of one's professional career, fulfilling the role of parenthood, children leaving home and becoming independent with their subsequent marriage and the establishment of their own families. Moreover, social and economic crises or achievements, as well as preparation for retirement, may be considered as some of these landmarks.

In contrast to the traditional psychoanalytic views which hold that middle age is a period of crisis, recent research studies find middle age to be one of the most fruitful periods of life.[17] Preparation for marriage and preoccupation with early marital life and child-bearing are over and most people have already established a career. Middle age, then, becomes a period in which caring and compassionate relationships can blossom. Generally speaking, many middle-aged people re-evaluate their lives and improve their relationships by expressing more love and understanding. The period of middle age relates to the 'generativity' stage of Erik Erikson's theory of the stages of life (these are: 1. basic trust v. basic mistrust; 2. autonomy v. shame and doubt; 3. initiative v. guilt; 4. industry v. inferiority; 5. identity v. role confusion; 6. intimacy v. isolation; 7. generativity v. stagnation; 8. ego integrity v. despair). It is a period in which one is primarily concerned with establishing and guiding the next generation.[18] It is in this period, when the nurturing attitude prevails, that contributions to the well-being of others become the hallmark of striving for personal growth. Some researchers[19] are of the opinion that, in this period of life, certain mature human defences, such as humour, creativity and altruism, will develop in response to anxiety and conflicts. However, development of such defences largely depends on earlier life style and personal growth.

The blossoming of caring and nurturing relationships during middle age is characterized, for example, by an increased involvement with the growth and development of children, seen in such activities as coaching youngsters in sports. It is also characteristic for middle-aged people to volunteer for humanitarian services and to take delight in serving a cause.

When one compares middle life with the adolescent period, one sees that the turmoil and unpredictability, competition and impulsiveness of adolescent life have faded away considerably by middle age, while wisdom and autonomy, as well as stability and compassion, have become prevalent features. However, those whose efforts to establish a career have been frustrated or who feel unfulfilled in their personal lives may not be as giving and nurturing as those whose earlier expectations have been met.

For women, the period of menopause may colour middle age. However, the behavioural changes that may occur will depend on the woman's personality, education, family environment and fund of knowledge about the process of menopause and transition. This is an area which still requires a great deal of research.

Challenges of Old Age

Towards the end of the period of middle age one begins to notice signs that another stage in life is about to begin. Some of these signs are a cause of concern to many. Among the serious challenges of this new stage, old age, are the decline of physical health and the possible susceptibility to certain diseases. One of these is dementia, particularly Alzheimer's disease, so frequently talked about in various parts of the world today. Increasing concern about this disease has prompted me to devote an entire chapter to this subject.

Creativity in Old Age

Getting old, however, should not be equated with sickness or uselessness. Ageing can be a very fulfilling and creative process. Old age is a period of freedom from the anxiety of occupational achievement and raising children. It can be a period of reflection on the meaning of life and the individual's place in the universe. As the person grows in wisdom, personal goals are directed towards inner reality. In this phase of existence the struggle to have is often overcome by the will to be.

In many people, the creative process unfolds with ageing. There are numerous examples of creative people who produced masterpieces of literary, scientific, artistic, philosophical or other work in old age. In the history of the Bahá'í Faith, too, a number of individuals have risen to prominence and service to the Bahá'í Cause in the latter part of their lives.

This book intends to address the process of ageing and coping in the light of the Bahá'í Writings and current professional knowledge. Old age is a neglected period of human life which needs to be closely examined, understood and prepared for.

1

Our Ageing Society:
Some Statistics and Reflections

Old age is the last of the evolutionary periods an individual passes through during the course of a lifetime. Like the periods or cycles of childhood and adolescence, this stage has a character and quality of its own. During this period the person fulfils a certain biological, psychological and spiritual potential. There has been very little research on the significance of this period because it is generally perceived to be the end of the journey of human life. But the final stage of this journey can be as exciting as the beginning, a landmark for the approach to the traveller's eternal home and a time to reflect upon and ponder over the entire journey.

'Young' and 'Old' as Symbols

The determination of what is young or old depends, to a large extent, not only on the biological aspect of ageing, but also on one's psychological impression of oneself. There is a general reluctance among women in western society to admit to the reality of ageing. This trend is rooted in the cultural idealization of youth and youthful attraction. However, as Levinson points out, the terms 'youth' and 'old age' also have other interpretations and meanings.[1]

In their fullest meaning, the terms 'young' and 'old' are not tied to specific age levels. They are symbols that refer to basic psychological, biological and social qualities of human life at every age ... We start becoming old at birth, just as we remain young in certain respects during old age.

Ultimately, 'young' is an archetypal symbol with many meanings. It represents birth, growth, possibility, initiation, openness, energy, potential. It colours the meaning we give to many concrete images: the infant, sunrise, the New Year, the seed, the blossoms and rites of spring, the newcomer, the promise, the vision of things to come. We are young at any age to the extent that these associations colour our psychological, biological and social functioning.

Conversely, 'old' is a symbol representing termination, fruition, stability, structure, completion, death. Its images include Father Time, the Grim Reaper, the Rock of Ages, the Wise Old Man, the dotard, winter, midnight. The immovable object of age confronts the irresistible force of youth ...

Being Young, like being Old, has advantages and disadvantages, strengths and limitations. Each state can be given positive as well as negative meanings. To be Young is to be lively, growing, heroic, full of possibilities; but it is also to be fragile, imperfectly developed, impulsive, lacking in experience and solidity. Similarly, the Old person (whatever his age) may be seen as wise, powerful, accomplished, 'able to hear the dictates of heaven' (Confucius) – but also as senile, tyrannical, impotent, unconnected to the life around him.

The Young/Old polarity – the splitting of Young and Old, and the effort to reintegrate them – is the polarity of human development. It is the basic polarity to be worked on in every developmental transition. The symbolization of being both Old and Young – of death and rebirth, destructuring and restructuring, mortality and immortality – is inherent in the very nature of a developmental transition. We feel Old in that a phase in our lives is coming to an end and must be permitted to pass. Yet we also feel Young, since the potential for a new period carries with it the qualities of rejuvenation and growth.[2]

It has been said,

> Old age begins and middle age ends
> the day your descendants outnumber your friends.[3]

From the demographic perspective, the United Nations defines a young society as one where the proportion of people over 60 is 4%, a mature society as one with between 4% and 7% in that age category, and an ageing society as one with 7% and above. As there is an unfortunate negativism associated with the phrase 'ageing society', those who affirm the importance of biomedical research might prefer the phrase 'longevity revolution'.[4]

The Rise of an Ageing Population

One of the most important social phenomena of the twentieth century is the rapid increase in the proportion of the population who are aged. In the seven centuries preceding this one, the average life expectancy rose very slowly. In 1200 life expectancy was approximately 30 years; it gradually rose to 45 years by 1880. The average age increased rapidly after that to the present 69.9 years for men and 77.6 years for women. The trend is one of continuous increase.[5] In the nineteenth century only a small proportion of the population lived beyond the age of 65. Today, almost 80% of the population can expect to live through most of their seventh decade of life.[6]

According to the United Nations, in 1950 it was estimated that there were approximately 200 million persons aged 60 and over throughout the world. By 1975 this number had risen to 350 million. The UN's projection for the year 2000 suggests that this number will increase to 590 million, while by the year 2025 it will rise to over 1100 million. This will be an increase of 224% in the 50-year span from 1975. During the same period the world's population is expected to increase from 4.1 billion to 8.2 billion, an increase of nearly 102%. It is therefore estimated that by the year 2025 about 23.7% of the world's population will be elderly. In 1975 it was reported that 52% of all individuals aged 60 or over lived in developing countries, and, if this trend continues, that percentage will increase to 72% by the year 2025.[7] As the proportion of aged people increases, the problem of caring for and coping with the elderly suffering from dementias such as Alzheimer's disease will be one of the greatest challenges facing medicine, public health and society at large.

It has been reported that in the United States 'in 1900 the average life expectancy was 47 years. Only 4 percent of the population was 65 years of age and over. Compared to today's rates, higher rates in maternal, childhood, and infant mortality contributed to the low life expectancy. Since then, socio-economic and health progress have made a vast difference, so that by 1979 the average life expectancy at birth was nearly 73 years.'[8]

Butler further noted that 'a marked difference exists between the life expectancies of men and women. In the United States, women outlive men by nearly 8 years from birth and by 4 years from age 65 . . . Looking at the marital situation of older people, one fact becomes strikingly clear. Most [older] men are married; most older women are widows. One finds at least three times as many widows as widowers. The imbalance of women versus men results from a combination of greater life expectancy and the fact that most women are younger than their husbands to begin with. This result represents one of the most poignant problems of the aged.'[9]

Dychtwald noted that 'according to the 1980 census, up to age 50, women and men are still approximately equal in number. However, between age 65 and 74 there are only 77 men for every 100 women; between age 75 and 84, the ratio drops to 50 men per 100 women; and among those aged 85 and older there are only 44 men per 100 women.'[10] It would not be surprising, therefore, to find women's issues becoming more prominent as the general population ages, as women will have a greater degree of representation in the elderly population. While these findings may not represent a fixed

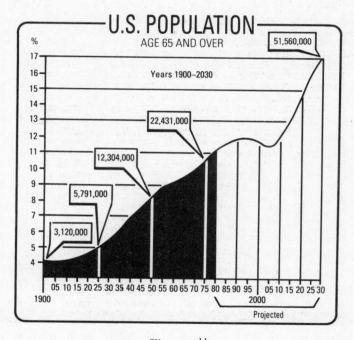

Figure 1[11]
From US Bureau of the Census, 1983.
Percentage of American population aged 65 and older from 1900 to 1975, with predictions for 1980 to 2030.

rate of longevity for males and females in human society, a parallel to this phenomenon exists in nature among certain species. In the case of bees, for example, the female has a greater longevity than the male.

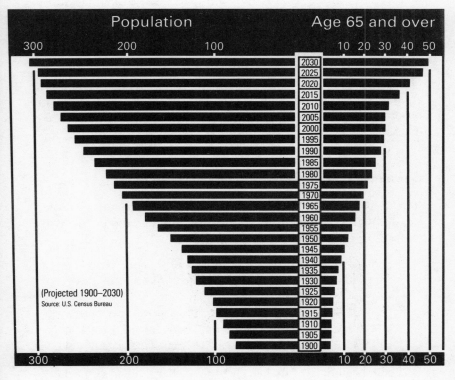

Figure 2^{12}
From US Bureau of the Census, 1983.
Bars show number of persons aged 65 and older compared with total population from 1900. The chart extends to the year 2030.

Factors Contributing to an 'Ageing Society'

A dramatic increase in the proportion of elderly people in society has been attributed to identifiable factors such as a decrease in the birth rate in industrialized countries on the one hand and the radical decline in the death rate on the other, resulting in a parallel increase of average life expectancy of the population. Infant mortality, natural disasters, and a host of infectious and other diseases have historically taken the lives of a large number of children and young people. With advances in science and medicine, a great number of these diseases have been successfully treated or prevented. On the other hand, problems associated with life style and stress, such as heart disease, cancer, stroke, accidents, alcoholism or other substance abuse, and cirrhosis of the liver and other diseases have become the major causes of death.[13]

Contemporary Ageing Society: A Demographic View

Basing his work on demographic data,[14] Robert Butler highlighted the following interesting points about the contemporary ageing society:

- 1983 was the first time in United States history that there were more individuals over the age of 65 than there were teenagers.
- The following example gives some perspective to the growth of population, particularly the ageing population. Japan's population has only recently reached 100 million. Altogether, 500 million people have lived in Japan since the beginning of its known history, 300 million up to the end of the nineteenth century and 200 million, or 40% of the total, during this century.
- There has been some success in family planning resulting in an overall slowing in the growth of the world population.

Growth over the past decade has fallen from 2% to 1.7% (1% in the United States). Nonetheless, at present rates of growth, there will be 10.5 billion people in the world in the year 2095 compared with 4.7 billion in 1990 and an expected 6.1 billion in the year 2000.

- The fall in birth rates has been accompanied by a fall in death rates: 19.7 per 1,000 population between 1950 and 1955 to 10.6 per 1,000 between 1980 and 1985 (in the United States the death rate was 8.6 per 1,000 in 1983).
- Europe's share of the world population has been reduced. By the year 2000 Europe will constitute 5% of the world's population compared with 7% today. Germany and Denmark are actually experiencing depopulation.
- Between 1982 and 2050 there will be a dramatic increase in the number of people aged 55 and above in the United States. One in three will be over 55; one in four over 65.
- The fastest growing age group in the world is the 85+ age group.[15] In the United States, for example, by the year 2050, there will be 16,000,000 people in that group alone. This is more than half the number over 65 in the United States today.[16]

Myths and Misconceptions about Ageing

The condescending remarks concerning old age which are often heard today are an indication of our stereotyped views on ageing. Many believe that old age is fraught with difficulties, characterized by loss, poverty and a sense of isolation and helplessness. The advertising industry and the media tend to ignore the elderly or to exploit and stereotype them. 'When older people take in this negative image of ageing, they cannot help but feel left out and worthless. The message comes through clearly: "You have to be young to be okay." '[17]

Theories about ageing and the art of longevity abound. One

ancient theory held that every cell in the body underwent important changes every seven years. Such years were called 'climacterics' because it was believed that they were years of crisis. A particularly crucial age was that of 63, called the 'grand climacteric'. This year, according to the theory, marked the beginning of old age.[18]

Dr Ken Dychtwald[19] identified several myths and misconceptions in present-day society concerning ageing and old age:

Old age sets in at age 65   There is no scientific proof and no biological or psychological event to mark a dramatic life transition on or around age 65 years. The figure 65 as a mark of old age and retirement originates from the time of Bismarck. In the 1880s Chancellor von Bismarck of Germany, in an effort to retire some of his military personnel, decided that age 65 was sufficiently advanced to be considered as an age for retirement. In an era when life expectancy was about 45 and 90% of the world's population could expect to die before reaching their 65th birthday, Bismarck's government chose this figure arbitrarily in order that only a few individuals would be eligible for pensions. Indeed, Bismarck knew nothing about human ageing and gerontology.

This arbitrary age for retirement was later widely used as a measure of the onset of old age and has been in force all over the world. In recent years, however, this age limit has been re-examined and revised as an age of retirement in some parts of the world. With the dramatic increase in life expectancy, age 65 is no longer considered a limit for old age and retirement. Rather, such a concept should receive a fresh look in the light of modern progress in health and well-being. As Dr James Paupst states, 'by taking away the right to "do" perhaps we have forced our older people to surrender their right to "be" '.[20]

Old age is like a disease In contrast to popular assumption, ageing is not a disease nor a handicap. There are many old people, past age 65, who are vibrant and enjoy a reasonable level of good health and vitality.

Old age brings feeblemindedness The popular myth of ageing being associated with feeblemindedness led many to fear senility as the expected outcome of ageing. 'The word "senility" has the same origin as the word "Senate"; both come from the Latin "sentex" meaning old. The root of the word connoted wisdom and experience, but in more recent years, it has come to be associated with mental degeneration and decline.'[21]

The other myths which Dychtwald has identified are that America has always been a youth-focused culture, that all old people are similar to each other, that all old people are poor, that old people are powerless, and that tomorrow's elderly will be very similar to today's older people.[22]

Robin Marantz Henig states: 'The old mind is like an old muscle: It must be used and challenged in order to function well. If housed within four empty walls and left to wither, the mind will indeed atrophy, roaming back into the past when it was put to good use and unable to snap back to the dreary present even when called upon to do so. But if enclosed in an environment that challenges, that stimulates, the mind not only will survive, it will grow.'[23]

2

The Psychobiological Clock

The human body is governed by a physiological system which is responsible for the measurement of time and the synchronization of internal processes in relation to daily events occurring in the environment. This system, which is also called the circadian timing system (from the Latin words *circa* meaning 'about' and *dies* meaning 'day'), works like a biological clock regulating biological rhythms. This occurs not only in human beings but in virtually every kind of animal and plant. The 24-hour sleep-wake cycle in human beings and the rhythms of reproduction are regulated by this biological clock.[1]

As we age, our biological clock alters these rhythms. For instance, the older we become, the fewer number of hours we spend sleeping. This phenomenon occurs irrespective of the light-dark periodicity of the environment.

Our psychological functioning on the other hand is more dependent on environment. A stressful environment will evoke one kind of response, a non-stressful environment another.[2] Psychological responses are influenced by biological rhythms and environmental stimulants. When our biological rhythms and psychological responses function in harmony, we cope or adapt well. When, for example, a woman accepts psychologically that she has reached the stage of menopause, a biological phenomenon, she is in harmony with herself and is better able to respond in a positive manner.

The ageing process, a lifelong dynamic force, is responsible for a number of biological and psychosocial changes. As age increases, these changes, including the cessation of specific functions, become more apparent.

Reproduction   'There is first and foremost the biological fact of termination of the reproductive function, an event that taxes severely the man's self esteem, so intimately related to his virile strength, and that of the woman, derived from her feminine attractiveness and female function.'[3]

Retirement   For both men and women, work is a symbol of contribution to society. People who stop working may feel that they are no longer making such a contribution. Because jobs usually bring people in contact with others, retirement from the work force may also lead to isolation and loneliness. Men, although they appear to be more independent, tend to be more isolated than women, who seem better able to establish intimate relationships with others and to adapt to the changes of old age.

Occupation may also provide a means for expressing one's higher and lower nature, closely related to positive and negative behaviour respectively. When the higher nature of a person expresses itself, love, mercy, honesty, fairness, trustworthiness, compassion and justice are the result. On the other hand, when the lower nature prevails, greed, jealousy, aggression and self-centredness are manifested. The implication of the closure of the professional outlet following retirement is that a person who has been working for years will, after retirement, stay at home with a spouse and possibly other family members. If the couple or family have not established a unified, meaningful and fulfilling relationship in the pre-retirement years, they could mirror to each other the expression of their lower natures, that is, they could behave in a negative manner towards one another.

Illness and Incapacity   Other changes occurring during old age are an increased potential to succumb to physical illness, the possibility of becoming incapacitated due to chronic diseases, and the decline of visual, auditory and other sensory faculties. Large numbers of elderly people suffer from chronic diseases, the most common of which are arthritis, hypertension, hearing impairment and heart disease.

Isolation   Separation from children and family is another feature of old age. During this period children usually leave home, if they have not already done so. In some families the offspring have already established their own families and have their own children. Therefore parents no longer have the same intimate contact of parenthood. A sense of isolation may be the result, coming at a time when many old people also lose their friends and relatives due to death or to relocation.

Perceptual Processes   Among other changes of a psychobiological nature in old age is a slowness in perceptual processes. The aged are less able to scan incoming stimuli and examine them in an optimal time period. Consequently, the old react less quickly than younger people to those stimuli. As Bibring indicated, an aged person 'is slowed down in his motor activities and cannot keep up with the pace of life around him. He is less dominated by his instinctual drives than is the young person, less emotionally involved in people and issues, less enthused about their virtues, and more tolerant of their shortcomings. He is forgetful and avoids as far as possible the barrage of incoming stimuli which renders him inattentive, but he is also less distracted and influenced by them. He is altogether more inner-directed than before, inclined to reminisce and to meditate. Whatever knowledge and experience he has acquired over many years and his command of intelligent task solution remain with him for indeterminate time ... His limitations lie in his increasing failure to remain an equal partner in the world of active striving, in his withdrawn and self-contained inclinations, and his lack of interest, attention and memory for outside signals and communications.'[4]

In the aged the remote memory is less affected than the recent memory. The RNA (ribonucleic acid), a chemical substance involved in cellular protein synthesis and thought to play a role in memory, increases significantly between the ages of 3 and 40 and declines rapidly after the age of 60.[5] This decline is probably responsible for memory loss.

Detachment A state of progressive detachment, resignation and renunciation of the world occurs.[6] According to the psychoanalytic theory of old age, regression to earlier stages of life characterizes this period. This notion, however, needs to be reassessed in light of current knowledge. The decline of libido and energy does not necessarily correlate with the decline of wisdom and understanding. On the contrary, many of the wishes, desires and dreams of a younger age may manifest themselves more freely in old age.[7] Like stars which are always present in the sky, they are not visible during the day but are seen shining at night. When making this comparison one may also recall that night is a time for reflection on the day which has passed and the day which is to come.

Environment and the Aged

Relocation from one environment to another, a stressful

experience at any age, can be traumatic for the elderly. Lieberman and Tobin[8] reported that of 639 elderly people (most of whom were institutionalized) who had changed their living arrangements through relocation elsewhere, half were either dead, physically impaired or had psychologically deteriorated one year later. In their study, the authors explored the conditions under which challenges to living space, loss and impending death are experienced as crises. They noted that individuals respond differently to stressful life events; some would flourish and grow, some would not be seriously affected, while others, who were unable to cope, would deteriorate psychologically and physically. It is not clear why some elderly people respond favourably to changes in the environment and others do not. Perhaps one of the reasons society fails to provide adequate information with regard to these issues is that the models which it uses to study the elderly are the young. The lives of the elderly have not been sufficiently explored on the basis of their own experience!

Tranquillity in Old Age

Peace and security during old age partly depend on the degree of inner serenity which the individual has developed over the years. The more dependent the individual is on the material world as a source of security, the more likely anxiety will be experienced and fear of anticipated or actual loss of that source will be felt. In contrast, if an inner peace and tranquillity has been established, the individual will be in a better position to maintain a sense of security in the face of the changes and challenges of the outside world. This inner peace and serenity cannot be attained and sustained without the help of divine education. It requires that one discover one's true self and attain a spiritual vision of the purpose of life. In the words of Bahá'u'lláh,

> Thou art My lamp and My light is in thee. Get thou from it thy radiance and seek none other than Me. For I have created thee rich and have bountifully shed My favour upon thee.[9]

3

Ageing and Creativity

In plants and animals ageing is associated with the cycles of the reproductive system. In some species the end of the reproductive cycle coincides with the termination of life.

Human life, like the life of nature, has a seasonal pattern of its own. This seasonal variation reveals new potential and brings changes. Each season is marked by the rise of certain human forces and the decline of others. Like each season of nature, each human season has its own beauty, its own colour and its own inherent qualities. Old age is one season in the process of human maturation and growth.

All created things have their degree, or stage, of maturity. The period of maturity in the life of a tree is the time of its fruit bearing. The maturity of a plant is the time of its blossoming and flower. The animal attains a stage of full growth and completeness, and in the human kingdom man reaches his maturity when the lights of intelligence have their greatest power and development.

From the beginning to the end of his life man passes through certain periods, or stages, each of which is marked by certain conditions peculiar to itself. For instance, during the period of childhood his conditions and requirements are characteristic of that degree of intelligence and capacity. After a time he enters the period of youth, in which his former conditions and needs are superseded by new requirements applicable to the advance in his degree. His faculties of observation are broadened and deepened; his intelligent capacities are trained and awakened; the limitations and environment of childhood no longer restrict his energies and accomplishments. At last he passes out of the period of youth and enters the stage, or station, of maturity, which necessitates another transformation and corresponding advance in his sphere of life activity. New powers and perceptions clothe him, teaching and training commensurate with his progression occupy his mind, special bounties and bestowals descend in proportion to his increased capacities, and his former period of youth and its conditions will no longer satisfy his matured view and vision.[1]

Ageing is perceived by people of some cultures as a kind of infirmity or sickness to be avoided at all costs, while in other cultures ageing connotes the acquisition of wisdom and honour. In countries of Southeast Asia, for instance, the elderly have traditionally enjoyed a privileged place in their society. They are respected and their advice is sought on diverse social and economic matters.[2] According to Dr Halfdan Mahler, former Director-General of the World Health Organization,

> Today, in many developing countries, there are still living customs which incorporate the elderly in the life of the community and these should be maintained. In fact, in these countries wisdom is still equated with age and the elderly are often considered to be the natural statesmen of the community.[3]

Dr Mahler maintains that the aged can contribute in many ways. For example, old people are particularly appreciated in the areas of art, sculpture and music. Another significant contribution of the elderly is their personal experience and presence which they share with those around them. For example, grandparents and elderly relatives play an important role in providing emotional contact for grandchildren whose parents may often be absent because of work commitments

and the like. They also impart to their grandchildren a body of
knowledge, wisdom and experience. In a similar manner
volunteer organizations such as R.S.V.P (Retired Seniors
Volunteer Programme) provide a means for the elderly to
share these precious gifts with a younger generation. (One
could also argue that their presence is often perceived as a
burden on society, but it is now felt that this attitude reflects a
selfish and archaic way of thinking.)

Paul Pruyser in his article on 'Creativity in Aging Persons'
indicates that the role and quality of aspirations change in old
age. An old person caught between remaining ambitions and
the anticipated loss of self may become aware of a feeling of
mournfulness regarding plans and activities. Furthermore, he
notes that the ambiguities of old age and the quality of
mourning over actual or anticipated losses may move some
old persons towards a late life creativity that may affirm any
past creative work or tendencies or may come as a surprise
both to themselves and to those who know them. Pruyser feels
that in old age people may think that they are running out of
time and may compensate for what they feel they have not
been able to do. He calls the aged people 'survivors' in a
special sense. In old age a previous rigidity of character may
be changed to a softening of earlier dogmatism and produce a
forgiving approach to one's own and others' shortcomings.
Pruyser concludes that the aged person, after becoming free
from the fetters of previous impediments and liberated from
the absolutes of the past, will achieve a sense of humour which
is probably one of the greatest forms of creativity within the
reach of ordinary people.[4]

'Ageing is not simply a physical process, but a state of
mind.'[5] Indeed, it is also a state of soul. In contrast to
common belief, creativity does not stop with ageing and in
certain cases may flourish in old age. Dychtwald noted that

some of the most creative minds of history produced their most gifted works in old age: 'Goethe completed *Faust* when he was over 80, and Humboldt worked out his great contribution to science, the *Kosmos*, from ages 76 to 90.'[6]

Michelangelo, a genius of creative art, lived 89 years. In the latter years of his life he was more involved with architecture, which did not require physical labour. He designed monuments for Rome such as the Capitoline Square and the dome of St Peter's Cathedral. Not only was he an artist and a sculptor but he was also a poet. In the latter years of his life, his poems were 'very direct religious statements suggesting prayers'. Michelangelo had a powerful sense of his own imperfection yet he was quite aware of the quality of his work.[7]

Another great Italian painter, Titian, was still at work at the age of 90 – and he was still developing his artistic style. In our own time, the Spanish artist Pablo Picasso, who died in 1973 at the age of 91, was still energetically at work in his last years.[8] Picasso, considered to be one of the greatest painters of the twentieth century, remained an innovator into the last decade of his life. In his later years, his work exhibited a renewed sense of play. For instance, he performed tricks with light and with brush and transformed paper cutouts into sculptures. In those years he also returned to his earlier paintings, re-painting them with variations.[9] In a way, one could say that he was summing up his life in a creative manner.

Composer Giuseppe Verdi was 74 when he wrote his great opera *Otello* and 80 when he wrote *Falstaff*, an opera full of intensity and humour.

The Chinese philosopher Confucius, who deeply influenced the civilizations of eastern Asia, continued to teach until his death in 479 BC at the age of 72.

Sir Winston Churchill, who did not become a world figure until his sixties, was appointed Britain's Prime Minister for the first time at the age of 65.

Jomo Kenyatta of Kenya became President when he was 71, holding that office until his death in 1978 at the age of 85.[10]

Mírzá Abu'l-Faḍl, the foremost scholar of the first century of the Bahá'í revelation, has left a tremendous treasury of writings and scholarly works. He spent the last ten years of his life in Egypt and was actively pursuing his research work and writing until the end of his life in his seventieth year. He wrote numerous treatises on the Bahá'í Faith and the Covenant of Bahá'u'lláh, and on proofs and prophecies of the Qu'rán and the Bible during those years. He travelled to the United States in the last five years of his life and gave numerous courses on the Bahá'í Faith in different parts of that country.[11]

At the age of 51 Tolstoy experienced a 'religious conversion', the result of a search for the purpose of life which he had undertaken from his youth. This conversion resulted in the formulation of his own kind of 'Christian anarchism', and his writings after this conversion reflect his new way of thinking. His major artistic work of this period of his life, *Resurrection*, was written at the age of 71.[12] It was around the same period in his life (from 1901 to his death) that he was in contact with the Bahá'ís and studied the Bahá'í Faith.[13]

Gandhi, who brought independence to the sub-continent of India and used passive resistance as a type of revolution, wanted to live to be 125 years old and, at the same time, to be active and fit. He believed that one could achieve this through 'right diet, mud packs, baths, regular sleep, internal irrigation when necessary, no alcohol and no stimulants – provided one also possessed the real key to longevity: "detachment of mind" '.[14]

Howard Colby Ives, a Bahá'í who was formerly a Unitarian minister and who wrote *Portals to Freedom*, suffered ill health all his life. Doctors predicted that he would not live beyond 25 years; yet, at the age of 67 he discovered that he had a gift for writing. Unfortunately, almost as soon as he began to write, his eyesight deteriorated. This, however, did not stop him; he learned to touch type. Mr Colby Ives had a very special attitude towards suffering. He looked upon his personal tragedies as bounties from God. 'When I recognize the undoubted fact that all this life has taught me . . . is but a sign, a token, a symbol, of what the future worlds of God shall surely teach – my whole being is lost in thanksgiving and praise of Him Who has bestowed on me – this boundless Gift and this infinite Bounty.'[15]

Siyyid Muṣṭafá Rúmí of Burma was an outstanding man and a Hand of the Cause (an individual charged with protecting the Bahá'í Faith and assisting in its growth and development) in the early days of the Bahá'í revelation. It is said of him that 'he was about 99 years of age at the time of his death but his spiritual being was as young or even younger than the spirit of a youth of 22 years. If he heard that there was an inquirer he would walk long distances and visit the inquiring soul . . .'[16]

Maria Montessori, the renowned educator and founder of the Montessori method, lived 81 years. During the war years, when she was well into her seventies, she spent her time helping with the establishment of Montessori schools in India. In 1946, when she was 76 years of age, a time when most of us are ready to 'close up shop', she turned her attention to a new area, the care of infants. After the war she travelled in Holland and England. Upon her arrival in England, instead of going straight to the house she had rented, she wanted to see the damage caused by the war first.

'Don't you want to rest first, Mammolina?' asked her hosts. 'Rest?' she said, staring at the two young women. 'What for?'

On 16 May 1952, a few months before her eighty-second birthday, Maria Montessori was seated in a garden in a Dutch village near the Hague, thinking about making a trip to Africa. It was suggested that because of her health she ought not to go but should let someone else give the lectures.

'Am I no longer of any use then?' she asked. An hour later she died of a cerebral haemorrhage.[17]

Eleanor Roosevelt, apart from being the wife of a President of the United States, was also a fine speaker and writer and a champion of human rights. She wrote two books, *Tomorrow is Now* and *You Learn By Living*, and was responsible for a question and answer page in *McCall's* magazine. In her seventies she participated in a television series entitled 'Prospects of Mankind', undertook university lecture tours and during the Kennedy administration served on government committees. A member of the Advisory Council of the Peace Corps, she also presided over the Commission on the Status of Women.

In her seventy-fifth year she wrote,

When you cease to make a contribution you begin to die. Therefore I think it a necessity to be doing something which you feel is helpful in order to grow old gracefully and contentedly.

I could not, at any age, be content to take my place in a corner by the fireside and simply look on. Life was meant to be lived. Curiosity must be kept alive. The fatal thing is the rejection. One must never, for whatever reason, turn his back on life.[18]

When he was 49 years old, Sigmund Freud wrote '. . . near

or about the age of fifty the elasticity of the mental processes, on which the treatment depends, is as a rule lacking'.[19] Yet there are many people who have passed the landmark of 50 the 'elasticity' of whose mental processes seem to be fine. If creativity is part of this 'elasticity' then Freud was himself a contradiction of his assertion since he was 81 years old when his work *Analysis Terminable and Interminable* was published.[20]

Ernest Strauss, an American mathematician who was an assistant to Einstein at Princeton University, once asked Einstein how ageing affected his thinking. 'His surprising answer was that he had as many new ideas as ever, but that it had become more difficult for him to decide which ones should be rejected and which ones were worth pursuing. In short, he thought that his nose had grown less certain.'[21]

Norman Cousins, the author of the well-known book *The Anatomy of an Illness*, speaks of his experience of meeting two elderly men of music whose creativity in old age he witnessed, namely Pablo Casals and Albert Schweitzer. About Pablo Casals he wrote,

> I met him for the first time at his home in Puerto Rico just a few weeks before his ninetieth birthday. I was fascinated by his daily routine. About 8 a.m. his lovely young wife Marta would help him to start the day. His various infirmities made it difficult for him to dress himself. Judging from his difficulty in walking and from the way he held his arms, I guessed he was suffering from rheumatoid arthritis. His emphysema was evident in his laboured breathing. He came into the living room on Marta's arm. He was badly stooped. His head was pitched forward and he walked with a shuffle. His hands were swollen and his fingers were clenched.
>
> Even before going to the breakfast table, Don Pablo went to the piano – which, I learned, was a daily ritual. He arranged himself with some difficulty on the piano bench, then with

discernible effort raised his swollen and clenched fingers above the keyboard.

I was not prepared for the miracle that was about to happen. The fingers slowly unlocked and reached toward the keys like the buds of a plant toward the sunlight. His back straightened. He seemed to breathe more freely. Now his fingers settled on the keys. Then came the opening bars of Bach's *Wohltemperierte Klavier*, played with great sensitivity and control. I had forgotten that Don Pablo had achieved proficiency on several musical instruments before he took up the cello. He hummed as he played, then said that Bach spoke to him here – and he placed his hand over his heart.

Then he plunged into a Brahms concerto and his fingers, now agile and powerful, raced across the keyboard with dazzling speed. His entire body seemed fused with the music; it was no longer stiff and shrunken but supple and graceful and completely freed of its arthritic coils.

. . . Twice in one day I [saw] the miracle. A man almost ninety, beset with the infirmities of old age, was able to cast off his afflictions, at least temporarily, because he knew he had something of overriding importance to do . . . It is doubtful whether any anti-inflammatory medication he would have taken would have been as powerful or as safe as the substances produced by the interaction of his mind and body.[22]

Albert Schweitzer is another colourful, creative figure who celebrated his old age with music, hard work in the service of mankind and remarkable humour. 'Albert Schweitzer', wrote Norman Cousins,

always believed that the best medicine for any illness he might have was the knowledge that he had a job to do, plus a good sense of humour. He once said that disease tended to leave him rather rapidly because it found so little hospitality inside his body.

The essence of Dr Schweitzer was purpose and creativity.

All his multiple skills and interests were energized by a torrential drive to use his mind and body. To observe him at work at his hospital in Lambarene was to see human purpose bordering on the supernatural. During an average day at the hospital, even after he turned ninety, he would attend to his duties at the clinic and make his rounds, do strenuous carpentry, move heavy crates of medicine, work on his correspondence (innumerable letters each day), give time to his unfinished manuscripts, and play the piano.

'I have no intention of dying,' he once told his staff, 'so long as I can do things. And if I do things, there is no need to die. So I will live a long, long time.'

And he did – until he was ninety-five.

Like his friend Pablo Casals, Albert Schweitzer would not allow a single day to pass without playing Bach. His favourite piece was the Toccata and Fugue in D Minor.

. . . The effect of the music was much the same on Schweitzer as it had been on Casals. He felt restored, regenerated, enhanced. When he stood up, there was no trace of a stoop. Music was his medicine.

But not the only medicine. There was also humour.

Albert Schweitzer employed humour as a form of equatorial therapy, a way of reducing the temperatures and the humidity and the tensions. His use of humour, in fact, was so artistic that one had the feeling he almost regarded it as a musical instrument.[23]

Positive emotions, such as love, affection, wit, humour and laughter have a constructive effect on health. Sir William Osler believed that laughter was 'the music of life'.[24] Norman Cousins was convinced that 'creativity, the will to live, hope, faith and love have biochemical significance and contribute strongly to healing and well-being'.[25] He wrote,

Scientific research has established the existence of endorphins in the human brain – a substance very much like morphine in its molecular structure and effects. It is the body's own anaesthesia and a relaxant and helps human beings to sustain pain. Exactly how the endorphins are activated and released into the bloodstream is not yet fully known. Nor is it known whether they might be activated by the positive emotions. But enough research has been done to indicate that those individuals with determination to overcome an illness tend to have a greater tolerance to severe pain than those who are morbidly apprehensive. Chinese medical scientists contend that the highly successful use of acupuncture instead of anaesthetic is made possible because the insertion of needles in the 'meridians' of the body activates the endorphins.[26]

The Value of the Elderly in Society

Ageing is not a life process we choose; rather, it is an inevitable law of nature. If we live long enough, all of us are bound to become old. Old age is an important stage in human development, not only for the elderly individual but for society as well. The elderly constitute a valuable segment of the human kingdom and possess a great deal of knowledge and experience in various areas of life. With their talents and their life experience, elderly people can serve as valuable resources for the children, youth and adult populations. For example, their knowledge and experience are important assets in the fields of organization, education, consultation, planning and counselling. Elderly people themselves gain self esteem and satisfaction by sharing and assisting younger generations.

For many ageing people, 'the third age', or the latter part of life, provides an excellent opportunity to fulfil one's potential. At the age of 81 Goethe wrote, 'My remaining days, I may now consider a free gift.'[27] Many now accept that

the special skills and talents of the elderly are valuable assets that can be used to the advantage of the remainder of society. It should be the duty and interest of the young and adult to assure that these talents and skills are fully utilized. There is need to incorporate older people into meaningful societal roles and establish a clear progression of occupational steps that one ascends with age ... The increasing number of educational associations and the success of the French and British 'University of the Third Age', catering to the elderly, is proof that the elderly are willing and able to learn.[28]

Social resources must be utilized in such a way that this age group can have an opportunity to continue a productive life. With this view in mind, certain experiments were conducted in the United States to stimulate productivity in the older generation. A number of programmes and activities have been launched for older people such as the 'Foster Grandparent Programme'. In this scheme elderly people spend 20 hours per week with a child who may be mentally retarded. 'Green Thumb' is another programme in which retired farmers participate and work towards the beautification of towns and the conservation of the environment. Those who are retired from business can participate in an organization called SCORE which gives advice and assistance to individuals who want to start their own businesses. Older people also find an opportunity to participate in the Peace Corps – an American-government-sponsored organization which provides volunteers to work with people of developing nations – or VISTA, its domestic counterpart.[29] Today many non-profit organizations and hospitals welcome the valuable contribution that elderly people can make. In the RSVP retired physicians, teachers, engineers, musicians, psychologists, businessmen and other professionals offer their accumulated experience and knowledge as advisors. Other organizations which mobilize the resources of the elderly are the American Association of

Retired Persons which provides valuable information concerning similar volunteer opportunities in the nation, the International Executive Service Corporation which places retired executives in small scale businesses in other countries, and the National Executive Service Corps which uses retired executives' expertise in domestic firms.[30] All these and other activities will help the elderly to feel useful and appreciated by society.

4

The Challenges of Old Age

Elderly people are faced with a number of challenges. Foremost among these are loneliness and a sense of isolation or abandonment. In many developing countries where the extended family is still preserved, aged people may feel relatively secure. In those societies where the nuclear family prevails and both husband and wife go out to work, this may not be the case. Widows and widowers are particularly susceptible to feelings of loneliness. The following vignette illustrates this sentiment.

> 'Grow old along with me! The best is yet to be.'
> The frail and crooked old lady slumped in the wheelchair is my great aunt. She is 83 years old, a widow. Her hands, once long and slender like my own, are blotchy, veined and knotted with arthritis. They are shaking so badly that I have to hold the book for her, open at the page where the above lines by poet Robert Browning appear.
> She reads slowly and jerkily, with obvious difficulty. Then I notice her gaze shift almost imperceptibly to some distant point in the visitors' lounge. She says nothing, but I know what she is thinking.
> She is remembering the husband of 61 years who died four years ago when he fell and hit his head against a park bench just a block from the nursing home, the children and grandchildren she hasn't seen since they made the trip from Montreal and Los Angeles last Christmas, and the cello she hasn't been able to play since her crippled joints forced her to give up a concert career almost 30 years ago.

Her eyes are moist and angry when she eventually turns
back to me. 'Poets – they're all fools,' she says. 'What he writes
there – it isn't true.'[1]

Attitudes towards the Elderly

The common perception of elderly people in any society
reflects, for the most part, the values most cherished in that
particular culture. In Eastern cultures both ageing and old
age have traditionally been viewed with a great deal of
respect. In societies where family bonds are strong and
tolerance is a virtue, where ageing is viewed as an expression
of accumulated wisdom, knowledge and life experience, old
people are revered and idealized as gifted mentors and
teachers.[2] There is a Chinese proverb which says that, 'if a
family has in its midst an old person, it possesses a jewel'.

This perception of old age, however, does not exist in all
other cultures. In societies where youth-worshipping, death-
denying attitudes are idealized, where worldly ambition,
strength and capability to dare and venture, compete and
change are the essential values of life, elderly people – who are
slow in their thinking, hesitant in their movement and
conservative in their attitudes – are either ignored or
tolerated, but they are not recognized as performing any
significant function or having any particular value.

Physical and Psychological Challenges of Old Age

Regardless of cultural differences, there are certain biological
and psychological changes which occur in all human beings as
they age which are of concern to the elderly and to their
families everywhere.

Dementia

Dementia, probably the most dreaded of all debilities, is a condition which is characterized by confusion, memory loss and disorientation. Although it occurs most frequently among the elderly, it is not considered to be an inevitable part of growing old. Only about 15% of those over 65 suffer serious mental impairment; half of these suffer from Alzheimer's disease. For much of the remainder, mental impairment from conditions such as heart disease, liver or thyroid dysfunction and dietary deficiency is either reversible or preventable.

It has been estimated that the number of people who will be affected by dementing diseases will rise substantially over the next several decades. However, it will be a gradual not an explosive increase. Some of these will be AIDS patients under the age of 65 who will develop dementia caused by viral infection of the brain. Unfortunately, persons with dementia are at particular risk of receiving substandard care, especially in an institution, because they cannot communicate effectively.[3]

The early symptoms of dementia have been described as follows:[4]

LOSSES   This group of symptoms includes memory impairment, decline in the ability to care for one's self and one's affairs and in work performance.

CHANGES IN BEHAVIOUR   Uncharacteristic behaviour, social withdrawal, personality and mood changes and paranoia.

ACUTE CONFUSION WHICH FAILS TO CLEAR WITHIN A REASONABLE PERIOD OF TIME   Behavioural crises may occur, such as being lost in the street, leaving the gas or water taps on, behaving in an uninhibited manner, shoplifting, forgetting to take medication or overdosing. These may be early symptoms of memory deterioration.

Depression

Depression, often mistaken for senility or dementia, is by far the single most ignored disorder among the elderly. About 15% of older people suffer from this condition. Major stresses, including the death of a spouse, are often the cause.[5] The symptoms of dementia may occur as a result of depression, resulting in pseudo dementia. Pseudo dementia resembles dementia but the symptoms are reversible. Very often a depressed elderly person may be misdiagnosed as being demented. However, as soon as the depression lifts, the confusion, forgetfulness and other related symptoms also disappear.

Substance Abuse

Nearly 80% of those 65 and over have at least one chronic illness (the top four being arthritis, high blood pressure, hearing impairment and heart disease). For these, the elderly in Western countries rely on a battery of over-the-counter or prescription drugs. The majority in this age group use more than five medications and 10% take over 12. Interactions among drugs, as well as too much of some drugs, can cause a host of complications, from mental confusion to slowed blood clotting to disturbance of the heart's rhythm.

Among the elderly, alcohol is the foremost substance of abuse, followed by drugs obtained legally through prescription and over the counter. About 10% of all alcoholics undergoing treatment are over 60 years of age. In Canada, in just four years, from 1969 to 1973, the death rate from the toxic effects of alcohol for women over the age of 60 rose 500%.[6] The death rate from alcohol combined with other drugs in the same group increased by 67%. Cirrhosis of the liver due to alcohol

abuse caused a 106% increase in deaths among men and
172% in women over an eight-year period, from 1965 to 1973.
The number of prescriptions written for those over the age of
55 in the United States totalled more than 225 million
annually by 1977; 80% of these were for mood-altering
drugs

Substance abuse in the elderly is often caused by distress
which needs to be diagnosed and treated. Many people are
unwilling to acknowledge the suicidal behaviour behind much
of senile alcoholism. Most elderly people were not brought up
to deal with their emotional problems and, in addition, they
consider alcoholism a sin. To confront substance abuse, they
must first confront their own fears and misconceptions about
growing old and then develop a healthy attitude towards
ageing as a natural and inevitable stage of life. Often elderly
individuals who have a problem of substance abuse need to
work through their feeling of loss. If efforts are focused solely
on the coping behaviour and not on the source of the
emotional stress, treatment will be less effective. On a positive
note, it has been observed that older individuals are more
likely to stay in therapy to complete treatment. The prognosis
for recovery, therefore, is favourable.[8]

Some Defence Mechanisms

The psychological defences of old age are basically the same
as at any other age. However, there are certain defences which
are peculiar to the elderly. In the psychoanalytic theory of
personality structure and psychic apparatus (mind) there are
essential elements: the id, the ego and the superego. The id is
described as the seat of the primitive desires and instinctual
drives. The superego is considered to be the moral equivalent
of the conscience. The development of superego takes place

during childhood through identification with moral figures, namely the parents and other role models. Through this process the child incorporates into his evolving conscience the values and moral precepts of his parents. Thus parents and other important figures in society become models for personality development. Religion and societal standards of ethics play an important role in the development of conscience. Consequently, the conscience may be characterized as being harsh, lenient or moderate and well-balanced. The ego (or self) is the executive mediator between the conscience and the instinctual forces and reality. (This term ego should not be confused with that which connotes egoism and selfishness.) It represents a number of mental mechanisms such as perception, memory and certain defence mechanisms. On the basis of these mechanisms it works to compromise between the unrefined and often unacceptable instinctual forces (sexual, aggressive, etc.) and the conscience, thus preventing psychological conflicts and personality crises (like a mediator between an unruly child and a prohibiting parent). When the ego or the mediator fails in its function, conflicts arise. In advanced age, the nature and expression of these conflicts may be to some extent different from other developmental periods partly because the intensity of instinctual drives is changing. But there are other conscious or unconscious desires and forces which may lead to conflicts.

Butler[9] identifies a number of defence mechanisms in the aged population. These are denial, regression, counterphobia, idealization, rigid personalities, selective memory, exclusion of stimuli, secondary gain, adaptive value of psychopathology, restitutive, replacement and compensatory behaviour, and use of activity. We will look at some of these in more detail.

Denial   As do individuals in other age groups, elderly people deny old age, i.e. 'This isn't happening to me.' Cosmetic surgeons can depict for you the profile of denial in the greying population of our time – the facelifts, the breast lifts, the eye lifts, the nose modifications, the tummy tucks, etc. Particularly in their 40s and 50s women (and also men) come to repair the ravages of time on their body by tightening the skin and muscles in the theatre of cosmetic surgery. By having a facelift they turn the clock back five or ten years and pretend that they are younger. In doing so they ignore the reality of ageing which is often related to death and dying. Denial is a common defence mechanism by which one does not acknowledge an internal or external reality. For example, a 60-year-old man is hospitalized for abdominal pain. After extensive evaluation he is told that he suffers from a cancer. He does not believe it and insists that it is indigestion and he should go home. He is terrified of death as a possible consequence and denies the reality of this illness.

Regression   In some individuals, facing the reality of old age is quite painful, and regression or return to the behaviour of an earlier stage of life becomes a psychological escape to the better days of the past. As a result, the aged person may become 'childish' or may present 'childlike' behaviour. Some are said to experience a 'second childhood' in old age. Regression is descending to a lower level of day to day functioning during which people feel unable to carry on adult responsibilities and expect others to take care of them as though they were disabled. Regression may occur in other life circumstances and as a result of physical or mental disorders.

Idealization   This is an over-estimation of an object, a person or a status. Elderly people may try to compensate for the loss of a spouse or a loved one by idealizing her or him. Idealization may concern an attractive job or position held in the past. Some people may experience this after their retirement. They overvalue the status they once enjoyed, write about it and praise it abundantly. Self-idealization occurs more frequently among younger age groups; older people tend to idealize others, particularly a lost spouse or grandchildren. The human mind is like a camera and the will is like the photographer. The more we turn this camera towards ourselves, our loved ones and our former positions, the more involved we become. To some extent this is normal but when the camera remains in the same place for too long, our perception of ourselves, for example, becomes excessive and our mind is no longer world-embracing.

Rigid personality   The behavioural rigidity observed in some elderly people is interpreted as a defence against the threats and insecurity of life; otherwise there is no clear indication that with the advancement of age one develops a rigid personality. For example, often elderly people show a rigid attitude towards their finances and how they are being handled. At times they may become mistrustful, if not paranoid about their money matters and financial management by relatives. This is partly understandable in light of the fact that with some exceptions, the majority of elderly people do not generate new income and have to be dependent on limited savings or income from their pensions. This threat of poverty and consequent homelessness becomes a cause of considerable fear and anxiety which would encourage rigidity as a way of self protection. In others, rigidity is a personality trait which they have had all their lives and which intensifies during later age.

Selective memory   Difficulty in remembering, particularly events of the recent past, has generally been attributed to senile brain disease in old age. However, in old age such selective 'forgetfulness' may be due to the fact that the person is avoiding certain memories which are too painful to acknowledge. For example, a seventy-year-old widow would frequently speak of happy events associated with raising her children and their travelling together with her late husband. Her face is animated when she speaks of family reunions and anniversaries, but she is distinctly silent about events which took place after her husband died two years earlier. The propensity of good old memories overshadowed her recent lonely life. Stressful life events can also affect memory and concentration.[10]

Exclusion of stimuli By blocking off certain stimuli, old people avoid those situations for which they are not prepared. Avoiding stressful stimuli is a protective measure to prevent painful consequences. A contrasting behavioural attitude is apparent among the young who are adventurous and seek out stimuli sometimes to an excessive degree.

Spiritual Responses to Old Age

Parallel to the psychological changes mentioned above, the spirit or soul of the individual also evolves. In many individuals, spiritual responses mature with ageing. In these individuals we may see expressions of a higher level of spiritual functioning which would override the more primitive psychological defences.

Denial The soul, which sees 'the end in the beginning', has no need to deny reality. Therefore, denial is counteracted with acknowledgement and faith as a response to the painful realities of life.

Idealization Since God is the object of worship and adoration of those who have recognized Him, idealization of persons or objects important in one's past does not occur. The person accepts these losses as expressions of God's Will.

Rigidity   Although there is, perhaps, no specific spiritual response to rigidity, the acquisition of such virtues as patience and forbearance, as well as reliance on God, enables a person to widen his vision and feel more secure.

Selective memory   For a believer, the source of knowledge is the knowledge of God and His remembrance. This belief enables one to rely on God and to acquiesce radiantly in His Will. The consciousness that the Supreme Will of God operates in human affairs makes it easier to accept those life events which are beyond our control.

Exclusion of stimuli   A spiritual vision of life permits stressful stimuli to be welcomed as challenges leading to further growth. In the words of Viktor Frankl: 'Suffering ceases to be suffering in some way at the moment it finds a meaning, such as the meaning of sacrifice.'[11] The meaning of suffering, when it comes to us unsolicited, is the meaning of the tender seedling bursting forth from its protective shell, sacrificing its essence to a greater end – the creation of a mighty oak.

Some Other Psychological Challenges of Old Age

Loss   Whether due to the death of a loved one or a friend or to a change in social status or material wealth, loss is a problem which commonly occurs in old age. Since older people are slower in adapting to stress and may experience more than one loss at a time, they invest a great deal of emotional and physical energy in grieving over losses.

Retirement   Men in particular find retirement difficult to accept as it involves not only loss of meaningful work, but also of the comradeship of friends and colleagues associated with work. Traditionally it was the man who would retire from his job and the woman who would manage the house. In some homes, however, after retirement, the man may take over the management of the household and dethrone the woman from her traditional role. This generates a great deal of frustration and resentment.

In recent years there has been an increasing number of women who have chosen careers in addition to their household tasks. More than 50% of families in North America are now dual career[12] – that is, both husbands and wives have jobs – and the number is on the increase. This emerging dual career family has forced the family members to re-examine their life style and to adopt a more reasonable and flexible relationship after retirement. In addition, more and more women, whether married or not, are joining the work force every year.

The issue of women and retirement has not been sufficiently researched, and reports are conflicting. Some researchers suggest that women adjust more rapidly to retirement than do men. Others indicate that due to a greater life expectancy and a longer retirement period, women face a greater challenge and hardship after retirement. Moreover, women are more likely to face this period alone, as their spouses often die before them. Their lower retirement income tends to make retired women poorer than retired men.[13] However, there are many exceptions to this trend, especially in countries where cultural attitudes and socio-economic factors are different from those in North America.

What is crucial in the post-retirement period is that the retired couple be able to communicate effectively and positively about their feelings and thoughts in replanning their lives. A marriage can be strengthened or break down depending on how much the couple empathize with and relate to each other lovingly as they follow the path of retirement.

Some couples will become more dependent on each other as

they retire since they can no longer depend on their children, who have often established themselves elsewhere. When one partner dies, leaving the other to cope alone, the surviving partner may transfer that dependency to the children. In this way the surviving spouse may be able to fulfil some of his or her needs.

In some cultures children are very receptive to these needs, while in others the children would rather see their elderly parents looked after by the government or other institutions. Elderly parents may sometimes exaggerate the physical and emotional symptoms of any illness they may have in order to legitimize and reinforce their need to be dependent on their children.

In some families the children may become abusive towards their elderly parents. Research in recent years has shown that where the offspring are involved in substance abuse and are under financial pressure, they are more likely to abuse their elderly parents, particularly if the parents are bedridden or suffer from chronic diseases which require constant nursing. Reports indicate that more elderly females than males are the subject of abuse, particularly after the age of 75.[14] These trends suggest that society should provide the older generation with financial and medical resources so that the security of the elderly will not depend solely on their children or on the limited incomes provided by their pensions.

Marital problems   Surprisingly, the occurrence of separation, divorce and sexual problems are high among the elderly.[15]

Loneliness   As stated in the preceding pages, loneliness is quite common in old age. As a result, alcoholism and suicide rates among the aged are higher than any other age group.

Loneliness can be particularly pronounced in individuals

who no longer work and who in the past over-valued their jobs and professions as a major source of satisfaction and security. An individual's conviction that his job is indispensable can render him vulnerable when that 'indispensable' source of satisfaction is no longer available. Loneliness and feelings of depression and despair may occur more frequently in those who have been forced into an early retirement and are unable to establish themselves in another job. Loss of a job and loss of contact with colleagues, or a sense of failure in being unable to keep up with the demands of an over-idealized job, may lead the person to feel unworthy and abandoned. The worst comes when emotional contact with loved ones is no longer available as a result of death or separation.

Some elderly people engage themselves in volunteer activities and find a solace and comfort in helping others. Some others rely on faith and ponder on the spiritual meaning of their destiny. Others will find the compounding effect of loneliness, poverty and abuses unbearable. They may seek an exit to this dilemma. Many may turn to alcohol or mood-altering drugs such as analgesics to numb their conscience and senses and to veil their feelings of despair and distress. Thus alcohol and tranquillizers become attractive options which are not too hard to find. The elderly may like this chemical excursion to the world of unreality and find in it a way to distance themselves from the cold and lonely world of reality.[16] Many become drug addicts or alcoholics. The adult children of alcoholics have a predisposition to heavy drinking and alcoholism. When depression and despair are too much to bear or to avoid even with alcohol or drugs, in some cases suicide may become a tragic outcome, especially if the community resources and support system are not available. Abuse of prescribed drugs in particular is quite prevalent in the aged population.

Decline of sexual function   There are many myths and misconceptions about sexuality in old age. One is that sexuality disappears with old age. Although there is a reduction in the physiological vigour of sexual functioning, sexual desire is often maintained throughout the ageing process with variable intensity. Life events, anxiety and stress of old age and diseases can adversely affect sexual desire and function. Men are more vulnerable in this respect because their failure to 'perform' is perceived as a reflection on their virility. Women are more concerned about their loss of attractiveness, but, on the other hand, after menopause the fear of being pregnant is gone. Physical and emotional illnesses further compound the fear of loss of sexual function. In a society where sex is overvalued or exaggerated as a basis of human relationships, middle-aged and elderly people may become very vulnerable to the fear of sexual failure. Yet sexuality has many dimensions of which sexual relationship is only one. The intimate and tender loving bodily contact of an ageing couple may provide sufficient emotional satisfaction which may be as fulfilling as sexual intercourse was at a younger age. Changes in sexual desire become more noticeable after the age of 50.[17] Research studies confirm the old saying 'use it or lose it', indicating that if a couple had an active sexual life in adult life they are more likely to continue this pattern with ageing.[18]

Rejection   This feeling is common among the elderly. They are very sensitive to the attitudes of family members and relatives because of their fear of abandonment. Consequently they will easily interpret certain events as evidence of rejection. Although sensitivity generally increases with ageing, it is related to individual personality and environment. It moreover depends on self-esteem and a feeling of being accepted with dignity. Reliance on faith is important. In cultures where older people are not appreciated the fear of abandonment and the emotional sensitivity towards rejection are greater. In contrast, in societies where there is a greater tolerance and a more positive attitude towards aged people, the elderly feel more secure. The personality profile of an individual, however, can play a vital role in the attitude of that individual and what he or she expects from others. Those who grew up with a rigid and mistrustful attitude towards others will be more likely to carry this manner with them into old age.

Fear of death Death is seen by many elderly people as annihilation. This concept of the finality of death may result in attempts to control death or to deny its presence. In the words of Socrates, 'No one knows with regard to death whether it is not really the greatest blessing that can happen to a man [or a woman], but people dread it as though they were certain that it is the greatest evil, and this ignorance, which thinks it knows what it does not, must surely be ignorance most culpable.'[19]

Elizabeth Kubler Ross in her book *The Process of Dying* proposes five stages of dying.[20] She believes that not only do these five stages frequently occur in a particular order but that they should occur in that order so that the dying person attains the final and adaptive stage. These stages are:

1. Denial and isolation

2. Anger and resentment

3. Bargaining and attempting to postpone

4. Depression and a sense of loss

5. Acceptance

Although a dying person may pass through these stages,

one does not necessarily have to follow this pattern. Rather, dying, like living, should be seen as a spiritual process. One does not have to have a certificate of competence to die properly. Nor are ageing and dying battles to be won. More correctly, they are physical and spiritual developmental processes which begin the day we are born (or even before).

We need to be open and to educate ourselves about this inevitable stage of the human journey. Death is a transformation from a material world to a spiritual world, a phenomenon likened by 'Abdu'l-Bahá to the transplanting of flowers in a garden:

> The inscrutable divine wisdom underlies such heart-rending occurrences. It is as if a kind gardener transfers a fresh and tender shrub from a narrow place to a vast region. This transference is not the cause of the withering, the waning or the destruction of that shrub, nay rather it makes it grow and thrive, acquire freshness and delicacy and attain verdure and fruition. This hidden secret is well-known to the gardener, while those souls who are unaware of this bounty suppose that the gardener in his anger and wrath has uprooted the shrub. But to those who are aware this concealed fact is manifest and this predestined decree considered a favour. Do not feel grieved and disconsolate therefore . . .[21]

In the Bahá'í Writings, death is viewed as an open door to a new world. Bahá'u'lláh states:

> O Son of the Supreme! I have made death a messenger of joy to thee. Wherefore dost thou grieve? I made the light to shed on thee its splendour. Why dost thou veil thyself therefrom?[22]

Thus the concepts of life after death and the evolution of the soul, when viewed in this manner, portray death as a final stage of human growth in this world and a stepping stone into the next worlds.

5

Coping with Stress*

Elderly people are more susceptible to high levels of stress for a number of reasons. Retired people often feel useless and this feeling is a cause of considerable stress. Moving away from one's own home into an apartment block, mobile home or nursing home, or becoming homeless, can cause an elderly person to feel abandoned by family and friends. In some cultures, loss of virility in men and attractiveness in women may further contribute to a sense of worthlessness. The decline of physical and, to some extent, intellectual ability is a reminder that being elderly may mean being unable to fulfil personal goals and objectives. The loss of strength and of the ability to defend oneself causes additional stress and insecurity. A great susceptibility to disease, particularly to physical illness, in advanced age may render some of the elderly helpless.

People need to be prepared for all of these eventualities in order to be able to cope with them and adapt to them in old age. The measures that can be taken which will enable a person to cope with the stress of old age will be examined later in this chapter. First, however, we will look at some of the

* Adapted from an article entitled 'Coping with Stress in a Changing World' by A-M. Ghadirian which originally appeared in *Herald of the South*, vol. 10, January 1987, pp. 34–8. By permission of the publishers.

general characteristics of stress, its causes and possible responses to it.

The Meaning of Stress

Psychological stress is one of the most pervasive phenomena of our time. It is a condition which occurs when there is a discrepancy between the demands made upon a person and his or her capability to respond to those demands.[1] Coping is a process which largely depends upon the human ability to understand environmental demands and to respond to them successfully. At a time of economic recession, political and environmental crises and social uncertainty, stress occurs as frequently as the common cold. Two-thirds of the visits to family physicians in North America are prompted by stress-related problems.

In recent years the term 'burnout' has become a fashionable expression in relation to stress and tedium. Burnout occurs as a result of prolonged exposure to work-related stress and is manifested by symptoms of emotional exhaustion and personal devaluation.[2]

Stress can affect people from all walks of life, but some individuals are, because of their occupations, exposed to greater degrees of stress than others. The staff of emergency wards and intensive care units, air traffic controllers, firemen, administrators and teachers, especially those working with handicapped children, are exposed to particularly high levels of stress. Now that computer technology is widespread in offices and even in homes, many believe that the increased sensory bombardment and emotional isolation which are often associated with working on computers may lead to undesirable emotional consequences.

Sometimes the circumstances of one's life may cause serious

stress. For example, the death of a spouse, which is more likely to occur in advanced age, is a major cause of severe stress. Divorce, separation, loss of another member of the family and loss of a job or retirement are other important sources of life stress. People who are members of an ethnic minority may suffer from the stress of prejudices directed against them because of the colour of their skin or socio-cultural differences. Being old and poor or homeless can be a very stressful experience which would further isolate the individual from others. Failure of sight and hearing and chronic illnesses of different types are other stressful life circumstances to come to terms with in old age.

Individual Responses to Stress

In any stress response and coping mechanism there are at least two basic elements involved: the person, and the source of stress and its intensity. A person's attitude towards stress and suffering will largely decide his or her future success in coping with it. If a person welcomes its presence as the 'spice of life'[3] and believes that without stress life is boring, such 'spice' may be needed! But if someone sees stress as a malignant virus which is about to attack, the person may have a hard time coping with it.

Psychological stress can originate from within the individual, as happens when there is internal conflict and prejudice. It may be caused by external events such as injustice, inflation, unemployment, social deprivation, atmospheric pollution and threat of nuclear war. Moreover, each person has certain needs which can be physical, emotional, social or spiritual. When any one of these needs is denied or frustrated, either unjustifiably or too frequently, the symptoms of stress will occur.

There are many factors which influence a person's perception of and response to stresses. Further, people differ in their abilities to respond and adapt to stress. What is stress for one individual may not be for another – and it may instead be perceived as a challenge.

The perception a person has of his environment as being stressful or threatening may be as important as the actual intensity and character of the threat itself. Linford Rees described a patient whose main complaint was an intense anxiety feeling. As the psychiatrist began to take a very lengthy history, the patient commented, 'I can tell you exactly what is the matter. It is my work which is the cause of my trouble.'

The therapist responded, 'Yes, tell me about it.'

The patient continued, 'I work in a fruit shop.'

'Yes, what do you actually do?'

'My job is to separate the large oranges from the small oranges.'

'Yes?' remarked the therapist.

'That's it,' the patient replied. 'It's decisions, decisions, decisions.'[4]

While the form and intensity of any behavioural response to stress will largely depend on the nature of that stress and on the individual's responses and cultural attitudes, various factors will influence a person's response to stress.

An individual's perception and interpretation of a crisis or threat will have an important bearing on the quality and extent of the reaction towards that threat. If one can make sense out of an event or crisis and draw some objective conclusion from it which would give new meaning to one's life, that stressful event may well be perceived as less threatening. For example, religion has given humanity certain explanations of events in life and history which otherwise could not be readily understood. These explanations enable us to make sense of and draw comfort from events which would otherwise cause great distress.

The following story illustrates how grief over the death of a loved one was changed into comfort by 'Abdu'l-Bahá.

One day 'Abdu'l-Bahá was asked by a woman if He would visit her sick child in 'Akká in the Holy Land. He came and brought two pink roses which He gave to the little one. Then, turning to the woman He said, with a voice full of love, 'You must be patient!'

> That evening the child passed away. When the mother asked 'Abdu'l-Bahá the reason, He said:
>
> 'There is a Garden of God. Human beings are trees growing in that Garden; Our Heavenly Father is the Gardener. When the Gardener sees a little tree in a place which is too small for its development, He prepares a suitable and more beautiful place where it may grow and bear fruit. Then He transplants that little tree. The other trees are surprised and say, "This was a lovely tree. Why did the Gardener uproot it?" Only the Divine Gardener knows the reason.
>
> 'You are weeping, but if you could see the beauty of the place where your child is, you would no longer be sad. She is now free, like a bird, and she is chanting divine, happy melodies.
>
> 'If you could see that sacred Garden yourself, you would not be content to remain here on earth. Yet, this is where your duty now lies.'[5]

This explanation of the meaning of death and the life which lies beyond it gave new vision to that mother and eased her sorrow. The death of her child became more meaningful and thus less painful.

Different individuals will respond differently to the same factors which cause stress (stressors). Responses will be both qualitatively and quantitatively different depending on the personality of each individual. For example, loss of one's job is a stress factor. Some people may become depressed while others may be moved to begin a new career. A person whose life has been characterized by passivity and resignation will have a different response from the one who reacts obsessively to the minute details of daily events. Similarly, those who harbour a sense of mistrust or even paranoia will react differently to threats compared with those who have achieved trusting relationships in life.

People experience stress differently. Stress due to ageing is a case in point. A person's birthday may be a source of joy or agony depending on the individual's expectation and what that anniversary represents. A woman who had just turned 37 years old came to me for treatment of depression. She was frustrated and enraged at a world which was 'unjust' and showed anger towards men who were 'insensitive'. She was a successful lawyer and held a respectable social position. But she was dissatisfied with herself and her job and felt that time was running out for her. During the course of treatment, she revealed a number of disappointments which she had encountered in her past relationships, all of which had failed to culminate in marriage. She was disturbed by the fact that she was turning 37, had not yet married and would soon arrive at the end of her child-bearing years. Each year her birthday represented in her eyes her inability to fulfil her dreams to become a wife and mother. To her, ageing was perceived as a road to an undisclosed destiny with no hope of fulfilment. In contrast to this is a 45-year-old woman, married, the mother of three school-aged children, and the bread-winner in a family because her husband is unemployed. She does not have time to worry about ageing! Her anxiety stems from her fear that she too may lose her job. For her, birthdays, her own and

those of other family members, are a source of joy and a
reason to celebrate. Ageing for her is a series of landmarks
along an eventful road, each day bringing its own challenges
and triumphs. These two examples of reactions to the stresses
of ageing highlight the fact that it is not only one's
circumstances in life but also one's attitude which determine
how ageing is perceived. In the first example, had this woman
found meaning and purpose in her work and accepted her
spiritual destiny, growing older would have been quite
different.

Societal Attitudes towards Stress

Society's beliefs, expectations and cultural values will have a
potent influence on the individual responses to life stress and
crisis. North American culture, as an example, values
competitive achievement as an important measure of success
and fulfilment. In such a society material success is highly
glorified while failure has become an index of guilt and
anxiety. Thus in a stressful situation, anything which threatens
individual performance becomes a source of dread and
anguish. Indeed, competition among college students is
reported to be not only the cause of major stressful experiences
but also a reason for their loneliness and isolation.[6]

Another characteristic of Western culture is the obsess-
ive pursuit of youthfulness, the attempt to remain young and
attractive. Women are valued for their beauty and youthful
appearance to such an extent that as they get older they feel
that they must hide their age and true appearance. Ageing itself
is despised and vigorously denied.

In societies where there is excessive emphasis on materialis-
tic attachments and material success as the main sources of

happiness, people may become more vulnerable to stress. Such attachments make separation from material excesses more difficult. Likewise, the more people become dependent on material power as a source of security and satisfaction, the more they will be susceptible to the stress of insecurity. On the other hand, if material power is subordinated to spiritual power, then humanity obtains greater security.

The advance of modern technology has changed our perception of the reality of stress and suffering. We now expect comfort and security in every facet of our lives. This, in turn, has made the task of coping with distress more difficult. With modern scientific discoveries, we experience an illusory sense of omnipotence and power to conquer the universe.

In such a climate, failure to master life circumstances becomes a new source of anxiety. Some events are so stressful as to be crises, beyond human control. Those individuals who feel compelled to control every aspect of life will thus find their task impossible. The incidence of alcoholism, drug abuse, suicide and violence in some societies may, in part, reflect this dilemma. The need for a certain degree of control over one's self and the environment is understandable and necessary but when this control grows excessive it becomes destructive.

In North American culture there are two contributing factors in the personality profile of stress-prone individuals: firstly, competition and achievement orientation at work and in society and, secondly, isolation and loneliness at home. We have already explored the prevailing evidence which substantiates the former. Regarding the latter, the disappearance of the traditional extended family on the one hand and, on the other, the appearance of television at home – which very often replaces intimate family relationships and further isolates the individual from his surroundings – will increase susceptibility to stress and tedium in a competitive world.

Stress and Personality

In recent years there has been some interest in exploring certain behavioural patterns which are implicated in the life style of stress-prone individuals. A major focus of these studies has been the relationship between coronary heart disease and behaviour that is competitive, hostile, impatient and time-urgent, known as Type A Behaviour. It has been noted that the stress of time-urgent behaviour, such as occurs when one is under the pressure of a deadline, raises the serum concentration of cholesterol. The rise of cholesterol and norepinephrine concentrations in the blood of Type A individuals contributes to a rise in blood pressure levels and, subsequently, to ischaemic heart disease.

Biological Responses to Stress

The human brain produces its own anxiety-inducing and anxiety-reducing substances. The latter are of special importance in coping with stress and suffering. The release of ACTH hormones and endorphins by the pituitary gland and other tissues is one way in which the body responds to the psychological and physical stresses. Endorphins are opiate-like hormones which exert an analgesic and calming effect and are considered to be the body's own tranquillizers. Migraine patients are reported to suffer from a deficiency of beta-endorphin.[7] There are indications that the practice of biofeedback, acupuncture and meditation will enhance the release of these substances. It is possible that in the future medicine will discover ways and means to turn these natural hormones on and off in order to alleviate pain and distress.

Excessive or continuous stress can shorten life expectancy by reducing the efficiency of the immune response, thus predisposing the body to various diseases. It may also inhibit the body's fight against cancer.[8] This may explain why there is a rise in mortality rates in the period immediately after the death of a spouse. During the grieving process it appears that the susceptibility to disease increases, possibly due to a decline in auto-immune efficiency.

How to Cope with Stress

The following list of mechanisms is designed to help the individual cope with some of the effects of excessive stress.

Acceptance of Stress

A certain amount of stress is unavoidable in daily life. A stress-free environment is a fairyland, unattainable and counter-productive in our world. To a certain point, stress is essential for individual progress and productivity. Stress is a non-specific demand on our body and mind which surrounds us even during our sleep. It becomes distress only when its presence is in excess. Even then it should be viewed in positive terms. 'Everything of importance in this world demands the close attention of its seeker. The one in pursuit of anything must undergo difficulties and hardships until the object in view is attained and the great success is obtained. This is the case of things pertaining to the world. How much higher is that which concerns the Supreme Concourse!'[9] 'Abdu'l-Bahá further explains, '. . . were it not for tests, genuine gold could not be distinguished from the counterfeit . . . were it not for tests, the intellects and faculties of the scholars in the great colleges would not be developed. Were it not for tests, the sparkling gems could not be known from worthless pebbles . . .'[10]

Recognize the Stress and its Symptoms

Have a clear and sensible understanding of a crisis and its contributing factors. Why is it happening now? How did it start? How can I cope with it? Some of the warning symptoms of stress are intestinal distress, rapid pulse, insomnia, persistent fatigue, irritability, nail biting, lack of concentration, increased use of alcohol and drugs, and hunger for sweets.[11]

Have a Realistic Attitude towards Stress and Coping

An individual's perception of and attitude towards stress and suffering can determine the outcome of his or her efforts to cope. Very often individuals facing critical stress resort to the defence mechanism of denial. One should acknowledge the reality of the crisis in question and look for a realistic and practical solution. Success in this task depends on accepting stress as a life challenge. Furthermore, coping depends on personal skill and capability in problem-solving and decision-making. A certain amount of stress is essential and unavoidable in life. Our attitude can make the difference. It has been noted that 'when a person faces a crisis . . . the manner most conducive to adequate coping is: (1) confront the crisis – recognize the realities; (2) confront the crisis in manageable doses – take respite as needed; (3) locate the facts – the unknown is more frightening than the known: (4) don't blame others; (5) accept help from others.'[12]

Reflect and Meditate

Reflection and meditation will give us an opportunity to reassess our life style and to recognize what has been happening. We need to evaluate our personal resources (physical, emotional, intellectual, social and spiritual) and regulate our responsibilities accordingly. There are times when we need to delegate certain responsibilities. We also need to reflect upon our lives and our responsibilities. 'One hour's reflection is preferable to seventy years of pious worship.'[13]

Will to Survive

Have the will to survive a crisis. 'Anybody can be happy in the state of comfort, ease, health, success, pleasure and joy,' wrote 'Abdu'l-Bahá, 'but if one will be happy and contented in the time of trouble, hardship and prevailing disease, it is the proof of nobility.'[14] Unless one really wants to overcome severe stress it may be a downhill struggle and little or no result will be achieved. Norman Cousins, author of *Anatomy of an Illness*, believes that 'the will to live is not a theoretical abstraction, but a physiological reality with therapeutic characteristics'.[15] Submitting one's will to the Will of God does not imply that one should stop all efforts deemed necessary to deal objectively with a crisis. Rather it means that when all efforts fail, one should recognize the wisdom of a Greater Will. The pledge of members in Alcoholics Anonymous is inspirational: 'God grant me the serenity to accept the things I cannot change, courage to change the things I can, and wisdom to know the difference.'[16]

Sports, Exercise and Relaxation

It is becoming increasingly evident that a certain amount of daily exercise is essential to maintain a healthy life regardless of age. Exercise is a practical antidote for stress. Although it does not solve the problem, it motivates and prepares people to cope better with stress and to acquire a positive attitude about themselves. It also breaks the cycle of strain incorporated into daily life. Special attention should be paid to personal health on all levels – physical, emotional and spiritual. Individuals, particularly those with Type A behaviour, tend to ignore the body's need for rest, relaxation and exercise. Premature ageing has been noted to have occurred in laboratory animals when they were exposed to excessive stress for a long period of time. The human body is like a delicate and highly complicated instrument which needs regular maintenance and care. This is particularly true in old age.

Nutrition

Nutrition plays an important role in coping with stress. Certain foods which would unduly stimulate the brain and cardiac function, such as spicy foods or those which irritate the digestive system, may need to be avoided or moderated. To overcome a sluggish start in the morning or fatigue during the day some people resort to coffee or alcohol. Today medical science recognizes that excessive consumption of caffeine may cause nervousness, irritability, hand tremors, insomnia, etc. The effect of alcohol is far more serious and the consumption of alcohol or any habit-forming or stimulating drug to overcome stress is a self-defeating coping mechanism.

Nutritional deficiency often makes coping with stress difficult in old age. Many elderly people, because of poverty, isolation or forms of deprivation, do not eat a well-balanced, adequate diet and consequently become depressed, irritable and confused or suffer medical consequences.

Moderation

The Bahá'í Faith teaches the observance of moderation, for 'if carried to excess, civilization will prove as prolific a source of evil as it had been of goodness when kept within the restraints of moderation'.[17] Many psychological and medical problems stem from excesses in nutrition and work habits, and neglect of sleep, personal hygiene and exercise. People who live in rich, industrialized countries are particularly prone to excesses of life style due to an abundance of material means and the competition to 'have more'. One's life style in such an environment can be very stressful. Moderation is the key to a healthier life.

One should try to moderate the load of responsibilities according to one's capability. Although an overload of external demands can be distressful, insufficient external stimuli and vocational activities may, likewise, lead to stressful experiences.[18]

The Healing Effect of Human Contact

Intimacy, friendship and personal contact with loved ones is an invaluable remedy for loneliness as well as for distress and despair. It is therefore crucial to establish personal bonds of friendship and contact. It is equally important to broaden this circle of personal ties with others to create a support system network, a system in which the individual gives and takes. To give and to care can be as comforting and reassuring as to receive and to be cared for. Having someone to love and with whom to share the joys and sorrows of life is an important factor in coping with stress. In times of crisis, an individual's need for affection and affiliation with others increases. The stronger the bond of love and unity among the members of a family or within a community, the greater will be the healing power at the time of crisis. On the other hand, isolation and lack of human contact may diminish the ability to cope and to resist stress.

The importance of personal contact and emotional support from others has been demonstrated by experimental research. Mice that were injected with cancer cells and then isolated developed tumours more rapidly than those which remained in contact with other mice. In clinical care units, patients who suffer from heart attacks have a greater chance of survival if they are visited by friends or relatives, or have a pet with them.[19]

Feeling Useful

When a feeling of worthlessness and uselessness prevails, people begin to doubt their reason for existence and thus are unable to face the stresses of life. Unless elderly people are totally incapacitated, there is always a way to make use of their talents, experiences and potential to do things which will make them realize they are worthwhile members of the family and community. It may, however, take some creative research to find an activity which will restore their confidence.

Having Faith

To have faith implies that one has patience and can accept difficulties, recognizing that they have a meaning. The spiritual power and strength to overcome adversities stems from one's own faith and conviction in God and in the Divine Manifestations. In the words of 'Abdu'l-Bahá, 'As ye have faith so shall your powers and blessings be.'[20]

Humour and Laughter

Humour and laughter are effective prescriptions for stress at any age. One of the misconceptions about ageing is the belief that the elderly lose their sense of humour. In fact, they have the ability, through laughter, to ignore what is impossible to change.

Laughter plays an important role in responding positively to stress. It is said that 'God loves laughter'.[21] Norman Cousins, in his efforts to overcome a painful and debilitating disease, resorted to the exercise of positive emotions such as laughter. With the help of his physician he collected comic films and humorous books which he used regularly in order to laugh his illness away: 'I made the joyous discovery that ten minutes of genuine belly laughter had an anaesthetic effect and would give me at least two hours of pain-free sleep. When the pain-killing effect of the laughter wore off, we would switch on the motion-picture projector again, and, not infrequently, it would lead to another pain-free sleep interval.'[22]

It is believed that positive emotions such as laughter have a therapeutic effect on the body chemistry. They stimulate the release of endorphins and improve the function of the immune system. Perhaps a link could be established between humorists, comedians and entertainers who make their audiences laugh and feel happy, and psychologists and psychiatrists who search to unravel the mystery of unhappiness. One of the problems of current psychological treatment is that the treatment environment is so sterile and devoid of humour that positive emotions are dampened while negative emotions are meticulously dissected and explored. Too much emphasis has been traditionally placed on cognitive interaction and little attention has been given to the expression of positive emotions.

'Abdu'l-Bahá loved laughter and His laughter was often a source of solace. He would laugh very heartily. While in Dublin, New Hampshire, 'Abdu'l-Bahá told an oriental tale to the audience and at its conclusion everyone laughed heartily. 'Abdu'l-Bahá went on to explain:

It is good to laugh. Laughter is a spiritual relaxation. When they were in prison . . . and under the utmost deprivation and difficulties, each of them at the close of day would relate the most ludicrous event which had happened. Sometimes it was a little difficult to find one but always they would laugh until the tears would run down their cheeks. Happiness . . . is never dependent upon material surroundings, otherwise how sad those years would have been. As it was they were always in the utmost state of joy and happiness.[23]

'Abdu'l-Bahá liked to see others happy. 'Be happy,' He would often say. On one occasion He said, 'My home is the home of peace. My home is the home of joy and delight. My home is the home of laughter and exultation. Whoever enters through the portals of this home must go out with gladsome heart.'[24]

Know Thyself

Identify one's own areas of weakness and strength. Recognize the early signs of stress and tedium and find a solution or seek out counselling. Depending on the nature and rigidity of job structure, there is a need for adequate rest or a break when pressure is too great. This pressure, however, may be more related to the lack of control over the circumstances of one's job rather than to the amount of actual work.

Excess in anything can be hazardous to one's health. Some people are unable to exercise moderation at work and consequently become 'workaholics'. These individuals find it difficult to enjoy leisure time and find it hard to take time off to relax. Vacations may be an ordeal and are perceived as a waste of time. Those individuals who have Type A personalities are often workaholics. When such a person retires from his job, he needs to make a major adjustment in order to come to terms with the reality that his regular occupation has ended.

One of the main factors behind workaholic behaviour is that constant performance (with or without perfectionism) becomes a way of fulfilment. Competitive societies encourage this type of life style. It can, however, be very taxing for the body and mind, and 'burnout' is a common outcome of workaholism.

Stimulate and reinforce any recreational interests that you have, e.g. artistic, musical or other personal interests, and keep this interest alive. Such pursuits will provide a cushion against the impact of stress and allow the body and mind to relax.

Service in the Community

Become involved in community activities and, as far as possible, as a participant and not just as an observer. The community should plan and organize activities with the elderly so that they will look forward to these periodic events. The Bahá'í community, with its special emphasis on mutual understanding and love for one another, can provide a supportive environment for both the young and the old. There is much to learn about the strength of this community relationship:

> Indeed the believers have not yet fully learned to draw on each other's love for strength and consolation in time of need. The Cause of God is endowed with tremendous powers, and the reason the believers do not gain more from it is because they have not yet learned to fully draw on these mighty forces of love and strength and harmony generated by the Faith.[25]

The Spiritual Dimension

Although closely related to the psychological adaptation to stress, the spiritual dimension of coping has its own unique qualities. The goal of the human soul is to achieve a greater perfection. The process of achieving perfection is independent of physical growth and development. Similarly, the experience of the joy and sorrow of the soul is independent of the physical body.[26] Therefore, the suffering and afflictions of the body will not affect the progress of the soul. Likewise, spiritual responses to stress differ from physical responses. Knowledge and love of God are twin pillars of the progress of the soul. When the soul is forced to deny its knowledge of its Creator, it loses its sense of purpose.

The spiritual responses to stress and crises are:

- greater reliance on personal faith and belief
- greater capacity to accept pain and suffering
- awareness of one's own helplessness and imperfection
- acknowledgement of a supreme source of might and perfection – the Creator
- reliance on prayer and meditation, and
- a heightened sense of purpose in life.

Shoghi Effendi stated in a letter written on his behalf:

We must not only be patient with others, infinitely patient! But also with our own poor selves, remembering that even the Prophets of God sometimes got tired and cried out in despair! . . . He urges you to persevere and add up your accomplishments, rather than to dwell on the dark side of things. Everyone's life has both a dark and bright side. The Master said: turn your back to the darkness and your face to Me.[27]

6

Alzheimer's Disease:
An Eclipse Before Sunset*

Consider how the human intellect develops and weakens, and
may at times come to naught, whereas the soul changeth not.
'Abdu'l-Bahá[1]

Alzheimer's disease, once called the 'disease of the century',[2]
is a type of dementia. It was first described in 1907 by a
German psychiatrist, Alois Alzheimer. According to the most
recent definition of the American Psychiatric Association, the
diagnosis of dementia is based on the presence of the following
symptoms:

1. Demonstrable evidence of impairment in short-term
   memory with inability to learn new information, and
   impairment in long-term memory with inability to
   recall information that was known in the past

2. Impairment in abstract thinking, characterized by the
   inability to find similarities and differences between
   related words and their meanings

3. Impaired judgement and disturbances of higher
   cortical (brain) function, and

4. Personality changes and disturbances that significantly interfere with work, usual social activities, or relationships with others.[3]

Due to the difficulty of establishing a precise diagnosis of Alzheimer's disease, its prevalence is not clearly known. However, the risk of its occurrence is age-related. It has been estimated that approximately 1% of the population is at risk of developing Alzheimer's disease by the age of 65 years. The risk of illness rises after age 65 to 5% and for those 80 years and older to 20%.[4] It is believed that Alzheimer's disease progresses more rapidly when it appears in younger people. In 1983 it was noted that 'about 2 million individuals suffer from Alzheimer's disease . . . ranking it as the fourth leading cause of death in the United States'.[5] A diagnosis of Alzheimer's disease indicates a 50% reduction in life expectancy.[6]

Biological Dimensions

A number of theories about the cause of Alzheimer's disease – viral infection, aluminium toxicity, chromosomal abnormalities, cerebrovascular amyloidosis, blood circulation, immunological deficiencies, and serotonin insufficiency and disregulation in the cholinergic system of the brain – have been proposed, but none has been proven. It is possible that the disease is not caused by a single factor but rather by a combination of factors or an accumulation of insults to the brain.

In the process of ageing there is a loss of the larger neurons (nerve cells) of the brain. (It has also been noted that the ageing of brain cells accelerates significantly with Alzheimer's disease.) In patients suffering from dementia, particularly of the Alzheimer type, there are numerous plaques of degenerated neuronal cells (neurofibrillary tangles) in the hippocampus and cortical regions of the brain. Differences in the symptoms of Alzheimer's disease are due to the appearance of these plaques either in the dominant or nondominant hemisphere of the brain.

Psychosocial Dimensions

While developments in science and technology have contributed to the rise of an ageing population, the question remains as to whether the human mind and soul are prepared to cope with all the physical, psychological, social and spiritual implications of this phenomenon. For instance, at a time when we are unravelling the mysteries of the universe and conquering nature, we face one of our worst fears – the fear of losing our intelligence and memory.

Loss of conscious awareness and the intellectual ability to appraise life circumstances and to maintain a dynamic and effective relationship with the world can be devastating, particularly at a time when, due to ageing, our physical, emotional and psychological strength is declining. The loss of the power of understanding presents itself like a monster at the end of the human journey or an eclipse before sunset.

The tragic impact of Alzheimer's disease affects not only the victim but also the relatives, who find a loved one slowly slipping into confusion and forgetfulness or turning into a mistrustful and belligerent 'stranger' in their midst. One patient with Alzheimer's disease was unable to remember that each night she would get up and go to the refrigerator for a snack. In the morning she would accuse others of stealing her food. For care-givers, living with such an individual is a test of tolerance and love, particularly if they do not know the vicissitudes of the illness.

Patients with Alzheimer's disease show their symptoms in

different ways according to their personality structure and the extent of their illness. They may interpret words literally, resulting in strange situations. One care-giver relates that her mother, who was 'house-sitting' while the family was away on vacation, did not close the car windows during a rainstorm. Rather, she had sat in the living room looking out at the car in the inclement weather. When asked why she had not closed the car windows, she replied, indignantly, that she had done exactly what they had requested – she had 'watched the car'.

When Alzheimer patients discover that they are losing their memory, a process over which they have no control, they may experience a sense of helplessness and despair. Following this stage they express considerable mistrust and anger – a protest against what they have lost. Loved ones can no longer be trusted and home is no longer home. In dealing with these symptoms it is important to assure the patients that they are not responsible for the loss of powers, but that they are responsible when they choose to blame others rather than acknowledge such a loss. As one care-giver told her mother, 'You have a choice, Mom. You can believe that you live with a mean and hateful person who deprives you of the information you need, or you can accept that you forget. There is no other explanation.' Two weeks before she died, the mother made a definite choice: 'No, I don't want to hate you,' she said. In her behaviour, she had made a similar response countless times; this was the only time when it was evident that she knew she was making the choice.[7]

At times patients may be totally confused and in some cases hallucinate and have delusions. They may bitterly complain of persecutions. They may speak to people who are not present and who, in fact, may have died years ago. They may mistake strangers for their relatives and reject some of their loved ones as total strangers. Their language of communication and their judgement will deteriorate and their tempers will flare up. Life becomes very lonesome as they withdraw into a state of total resignation and progressively slip into the dark world of oblivion. At times lucidity, presence of mind and memory reappear but, like the rays of the sun piercing through a dense cloud, they are sparse and momentary. As the illness progresses patients eventually move towards a vegetative life in which they become entirely dependent on others for their survival.

People with Alzheimer's disease are very sensitive to rejection; in fact, symptoms of mistrustfulness may serve as a defence against rejection. Although the memory is impoverished and judgement impaired, emotion is often present. As a result of fear of loss of control over themselves and their possessions, demented patients may decide to protect their belongings by hiding them. When they fail to find what they have hidden, they suspect others, usually the closest relative or friend, as the culprit. It is very painful for a loved one to be accused of wrong-doing and yet maintain a loving relationship with such a patient. But this is the very challenge that family members and care-givers face, as most of these suspicions are consequences of memory loss and symptoms of the illness.

Spiritual Dimensions

Although patients with Alzheimer's disease lose their memory and intellectual faculties, they often maintain a sense of intuition and a mysterious spiritual awareness. This awareness, which they are unable to articulate and express, transcends the barrier of their illness. Some patients, for instance, manifest a sense of humour even to the last moments of their lives. 'An hour before she died,' an Alzheimer patient's daughter writes, 'my mother ate some toast and drank some coffee. She thought she was in a library (she never knew where she was) and wondered why her bed was there and whether she would be allowed to stay. "Mom, you know you are not in a library. See! These are your pictures on the walls." We laughed. I told her that her granddaughter had called the night before, and she expressed her delight in, and love for, her grandchildren. An hour later she was gone – even at the end she still had the powers of love and laughter. Even the doctor was surprised at the suddenness of death; it was a gift.'[8]

In the Bahá'í Writings, special emphasis has been put on the human spirit as a 'Divine Trust'. According to 'Abdu'l-Bahá, this Divine Trust 'must traverse all conditions, for its passage and movement through the conditions of existence will be the means of its acquiring perfections'.[9] Furthermore, 'Abdu'l-Bahá indicates that the 'temple of man is like unto a mirror, his soul is as the sun, and his mental faculties even as the rays that emanate from that source of light. The ray may cease to fall upon the mirror, but it can in no wise be dissociated from the sun'.[10] From this remark we can conclude that if mental faculties such as intelligence and memory (like the rays of the sun) become impaired, this by no means indicates that the soul has ceased to function; rather it means that the instrument (the brain or the mirror) is unable to reflect the power of those faculties. Explained another way, if the computer breaks down, it is not an indication that the programmer has ceased to exist.

In the Bahá'í teachings the relationship between mental illness and the human spirit is like the relationship between the cloud and the sun. Bahá'u'lláh states:

Consider . . . the sun when it is completely hidden behind the clouds. Though the earth is still illumined with its light, yet the measure of light which it receiveth is considerably reduced.

Not until the clouds have dispersed, can the sun shine again in the plenitude of its glory. Neither the presence of the cloud nor its absence can, in any way, affect the inherent splendour of the sun. The soul of man is the sun by which his body is illumined, and from which it draweth its sustenance, and should be so regarded.[11]

As the cloud prevents the sun from illuminating the earth, likewise mental illness prevents the soul from showing its power through the instrument of the body. The movement or the density of the clouds will have no effect on the natural quality of the sun which is to shine. Likewise, the spirit, 'Abdu'l-Bahá explains, is changeless and indestructible.[12]

Know thou that the soul of man is exalted above, and is independent of all infirmities of body or mind. That a sick person showeth signs of weakness is due to the hindrances that interpose themselves between his soul and his body, for the soul itself remaineth unaffected by any bodily ailments.[13]

Therefore, mental and physical illnesses have no bearing on the progress of the human spirit. The spirit will continue to advance, as progress is one of the essential qualities of the human spirit. Thus a person may suffer from mental or neurological illness and yet maintain an inherent spiritual capacity.

There are certain misunderstandings concerning the relationship between spirituality and human involvement in life crisis and environmental stress. One of these is the assumption that 'being more spiritual' means having fewer problems to deal with or having no problems at all. A spiritual person has to face as many problems as anyone else but the capacity for tolerance and the ability to accept stressful life events grows with this vision of life. It is similar to a traveller on a long journey who realizes that there might be unexpected surprises, such as changes in climate, hazards of the road or unfriendly encounters, and who understands that new adaptations will have to be made if he is to arrive at his destination. This individual will accept crises as new challenges for personal growth.

Intelligence and Understanding

'Abdu'l-Bahá explains that 'the reality of man is his thought, not his material body. The thought force and the animal force are partners.'[14] He also describes the power of understanding as 'God's greatest gift to man'. By understanding is meant the 'power by which man acquires his knowledge of the several kingdoms of creation, and of various stages of existence, as well as of much which is invisible'. Intellect or understanding 'is, in truth, the most precious gift bestowed upon man by the divine bounty. Man alone, among created beings, has this wonderful power'.[15]

> Like the animal, man possesses the faculties of the senses, is subject to heat, cold, hunger, thirst, etc.; unlike the animal, man has a rational soul, the human intelligence.
>
> This intelligence of man is the intermediary between his body and his spirit.
>
> When man allows the spirit, through his soul, to enlighten his understanding, then does he contain all creation; because man, being the culmination of all that went before and thus superior to all previous evolutions, contains all the lower world within himself. Illumined by the spirit through the instrumentality of the soul, man's radiant intelligence makes him the crowning-point of creation.[16]

In His Tablet to Dr August Forel, 'Abdu'l-Bahá explains:

Now concerning mental faculties, they are in truth of the

inherent properties of the soul, even as the radiation of light is the essential property of the sun. The rays of the sun are renewed but the sun itself is ever the same and unchanged. Consider how the human intellect develops and weakens, and may at times come to naught, whereas the soul changeth not. For the mind to manifest itself, the human body must be whole; and a sound mind cannot be but in a sound body, whereas the soul dependeth not upon the body. It is through the power of the soul that the mind comprehendeth, imagineth and exerteth its influence, whilst the soul is a power that is free.[17]

Mental Illness and the Soul

In response to a query about mental illness, the Guardian of the Bahá'í Faith explained:

You must always remember, no matter how much you or others may be afflicted with mental troubles and the crushing environment of these State Institutions, that your spirit is healthy, near to our Beloved, and will in the next world enjoy a happy and normal state of soul.[18]

It is very hard to be subject to any illness, particularly a mental one. However, we must always remember these illnesses have nothing to do with our spirit or our inner relation to God. It is a great pity that as yet so little is really known of the mind, its workings and the illnesses that afflict it; no doubt, as the world becomes more spiritually minded and scientists understand the true nature of man, more humane and permanent cures for mental diseases will be found.[19]

Caring Attitude

Our attitude towards suffering plays an important role in our way of caring for demented patients. In a world in which suffering is to be avoided at all costs, caring for old and ageing patients with dementia problems is quite a challenge. Our attitude is the fruit of our knowledge and understanding. When that knowledge is enlightened with spiritual wisdom and the creative words of divine revelation, it can transform our hearts and change our character. One's attitude towards a sick person is closely related to one's understanding of the spiritual nature of that human being. If our understanding is of a material nature, our judgement is more likely to be influenced by appearance, status and wealth or other material concerns. Consequently, based on such an appraisal, we may lose or gain interest in caring for the person. However, if our perception of that person is of a spiritual nature, our judgement is not conditional; our attitude becomes one of universal acceptance. Moreover, we also realize that beyond the cloud of illusions and confusion of a demented patient there is a noble being searching to find its own destiny.

The Bahá'í approach to health and healing is reflected in some of the prayers of the Bahá'í Faith. For example, Bahá'u'lláh in one of the prayers says, 'She is sick, O my God, and hath entered beneath the shadow of the Tree of Thy healing; afflicted, and hath fled to the City of Thy protection; diseased, and hath sought the Fountainhead of Thy favours; sorely vexed, and hath hasted to attain the Wellspring of Thy tranquillity . . .'[20] The 'Tree of healing', the 'City of protection' and the 'Fountainhead of God's favour' are some of God's spiritual refuges, the understanding of which is beyond our current medical knowledge and perception and can only be attained through prayer and meditation. It also indicates that the ultimate source of healing, tranquillity and protection rests within the power of God's Will.

Family Observations of Alzheimer Patients

The changes that occur in a family with an Alzheimer patient are in some respects similar to, and in other respects different from, the changes which take place in a family where a new child is born. Both the new child and the Alzheimer patient need others to take care of them and both are helpless in many respects. However, the former will grow more and more independent while the latter becomes more and more dependent. When a new child is born into a family, the members usually respond with excitement and joy. They change their lives and make sacrifices in order to meet the needs of the new child. As the child grows, the parents gradually relinquish control, encouraging an increased independence until the individual passes from adolescence to adulthood and establishes a separate life. In a family with an Alzheimer patient, on the other hand, as time passes the patient becomes more and more dependent and helpless, ultimately requiring constant care. Consequently, families who have an Alzheimer patient have to give up more and more of their freedom and restrict their lives in order to accommodate the ever-increasing needs of the patient.

To cope with the symptoms of Alzheimer's, care-givers resort to different strategies. In one case, a husband believed that the cause of his wife's memory loss was physical and that she was not making adequate effort to overcome this problem. As a result, he decided that the best way to help his wife was to push her to do certain memory exercises to improve her memory. The husband would repeatedly quiz his wife about the names of people they knew or things they used to deal with and, if she had trouble recalling this information, he would push her harder, thinking that this would be the way that he could improve her memory. Instead, she would get frustrated and angry and would feel helpless. The misconception here was that the husband did not realize that he could not correct the memory loss, caused by the damage of brain cells, through repeating certain verbal exercises. He could, however, provide a great deal of help to his wife by reminding her of people's names and of other information whenever necessary. When the husband corrected his misconception and began to provide more positive help to his wife, her attitude changed and she reacted more positively. He, too, was less frustrated in dealing with her.

Steven Zarit and associates summarized some of the common problems reported by the family and other caregivers, including how behaviour is often subjectively interpreted as well as how it should be viewed as a result of the patient's loss of memory. (*See Table overleaf*)

The following case illustrates that providing too many choices may confuse a patient whose memory is failing: 'One man reported that his wife could not get dressed. But when the counsellor questioned him about the situation, it turned out she had too many outfits to choose from and mixed them all up. He found that he could select an outfit for her and lay it out, and she would dress herself.'[21]

As decision-making becomes more difficult, the best way to cope is to simplify daily life so that the patient will not get confused.

Another difficulty that will manifest itself with Alzheimer's disease is due to the changes in character and behaviour which occur during the illness. Patients who were very courteous, well-mannered and in some cases very inhibited may become quite belligerent, discourteous and uninhibited in language and behaviour. Among the most embarrassing is loss of sexual control which can occur particularly among male patients. Very often patients are not aware of the social and ethical implications of what they are doing and if the families are unaware of this loss of proper judgement, they may accuse the patient of deliberately trying to dishonour or

Common Problems Reported by Families Viewed as the Result of Memory Loss[22]

Problem	Typical Interpretations	Interpretation When Viewed as Part of Memory Loss
Asking repetitive questions.	It is done to annoy me, attract attention. Patient could control it.	Patient cannot remember asking questions or no longer has appropriate skills to get attention.
Patient is not aware of memory loss, denies it.	Patient should remember, why won't he face it?	Patient cannot remember he cannot remember.
Patient does not try to remember.	Patient is lazy, laziness causes the forgetting.	Some stimulation of memory may be helpful; patients may not be able to do this by themselves; if they become frustrated, it should be stopped.
Accusations (e.g. stealing).	Patient is crazy, just trying to hurt me. Patient does it to embarrass me.	This is one way of dealing with the insecurity caused by not being able to remember.
Lowered inhibitions.	Patient is trying to hurt me; patient should be able to behave himself; he does it to embarrass me.	The brain damage often causes a loss of control.
Memory fluctuates from day to day.	Patient is not trying; patient is only remembering what he wants.	Some fluctuation in memory is normal. Fluctuation is not related to a lack of effort on the patient's part. It is important to take advantage of 'good days'.

embarrass the family members. This issue of sexual disinhibition can be a very sensitive topic which requires careful and effective intervention. If it is not properly understood and handled wisely, it may leave the scars of serious traumatic experiences in the family.

Alzheimer patients experience not only fewer behavioural inhibitions but also disturbances of reality testing and proper judgement. In fact, they may show symptoms of paranoia. Family members frequently complain of erroneous accusations levelled by Alzheimer patients against their loved ones. Family members need to be reassured with a few words of sympathy, expressing one's understanding of how difficult it is for close family members not to be trusted. This may have a soothing effect and will let them know that others can understand their feelings of hurt and rejection.

Zarit and his co-workers suggest that the patients also be given verbal and physical expressions of affection. They noted that with these expressions of love and affection the tendency of patients to repeat themselves or become frustrated and restless is alleviated as they feel more secure and accepted. It is to be kept in mind that there is a substantial fear of abandonment in these patients.

In another case it was reported that a woman who was caring for her sick husband one night noticed that he was staring off into space. 'When she asked what he was doing, he said, "Watching TV." She started to get upset as she had in the past, thinking, "Oh, this poor man, how terrible." But she caught herself, and thought instead, "At least he's happy," and walked off to do something else.'[23] This case suggests that there are times when we ought to accept certain strange behavioural changes as long as they do not present a danger to the patient or to others.

Many researchers in the field recommend that care-givers keep a record of their patients' behaviour so that they know how the events take place and how they can prevent or manage a problem. Memory aids and reminders based on these records will prevent excessive frustrations. For example, in one case where a patient was suffering from advanced Alzheimer's, the husband noted that his wife would wake up very early every morning and would go to the kitchen intending to prepare a meal. Observing this repeated behaviour and being mindful of the possible danger because of her confusion, the husband decided to lock the kitchen door and take all safety measures for her protection. As a result, the wife would still get up and go to the kitchen but, finding the kitchen door locked, she would stand quietly there – probably assuming that it was not yet time for breakfast – until her husband would come and open the door. However, as the disease progresses, even such limited perception may be lost, thus making control more difficult.

Caring for Patients with Alzheimer's Disease: A Family Challenge

The most formidable challenge facing the family is to accept the reality of the illness, that it exists, that it has struck a loved one, and that it will persist until the end of the victim's life unless medicine discovers a cure. Because there is no cure for Alzheimer's disease at present, long-term care of these patients is a major challenge for family members or other care-givers who must deal with such symptoms as loss of memory, self-neglect, restlessness, dependency, confusion, depression, incontinence, falls and rage, among others.

It has been reported that approximately one third of those caring for patients with Alzheimer's disease themselves suffer

from exhaustion and stress as well as from injuries sustained
as a result of the physical task of caring for these patients.[24]
Mistrustful behaviour stemming from an altered perception of
situations adds to the problem. 'My greatest problem as the
primary care-giver', writes one woman, 'was not only exhaustion
but also the total absence of privacy. My mother was very
suspicious of any conversation I had with anyone, so she
would sneak around, listening in to visitors and telephone
conversations, always assuming that she was the subject being
discussed, and usually totally misinterpreting what was being
said. I thought I would go round the bend!'[25]

One of the symptoms of dementia which irritates care-
givers is the repetition of questions. One care-giver discovered
that there are two kinds of repetition: one which needs simply
to be accepted like 'red spots with measles' and another which
is characterized by rapid repetitions over a short period of
time. The latter type of repetition points to a deeper need
which the patient wants to fulfil. 'I discovered that if my
mother repeated the same question over and over in quick
succession, it meant that there was something which was
troubling her. It was usually not easy to figure out what the
real need was. It required an investigative approach.'
Realizing that her mother would not remember her previous
responses, each time she repeated her question the daughter
would respond in a different way, trying to get at the
underlying trouble. When she finally discovered it, which was
obvious from the mother's response, the question was never
asked again. The problem had been resolved.[26]

In caring for patients with Alzheimer's disease, as in any
other case of dementia, one should look beyond the person
who is mentally impaired and confused. According to 'Abdu'l-
Bahá, the mind is circumscribed but the soul is limitless.
Care-givers should reach for that limitless soul. As the patient

becomes increasingly inaccessible through verbal communication, greater effort should be made to establish and maintain a contact with his or her feelings and soul. But how do we know if we are in touch with the feelings of someone who cannot respond adequately to a question? How can we reach a person's soul when that person despises us as a stranger, not to be trusted? This is a most difficult challenge, particularly in the Western world where emphasis is placed more on the mind and intellect than on feeling and intuition. People do not know how to relate to one another through their souls, fearing that they may be accused of being superstitious. Spiritual contact through prayer and meditation and by the unconditional love and affection shown by family and friends will facilitate the contact these patients need, a contact which becomes increasingly necessary when verbal communication becomes meaningless or impossible. If the care-givers make a new adjustment to the needs of the patient, a new journey can begin. An example of such an adjustment is found in the following remarks of one care-giver:

> I learned to distinguish, much more readily, the essential from the non-essential, the primary from the secondary. 'Now' became, for my mother, an island of time with all its own needs: what I had done for her yesterday, or even an hour ago, became irrelevant. It is an incredible discipline which leads to an important truth: nobody flourishes well on yesterday's love just as yesterday's sun yields no tan, and yesterday's meals assuage no hunger. Memory is wonderful, but it is no substitute for making good use of 'now'.[27]

Often family members and care-givers of an Alzheimer patient are frustrated because they are concerned with the 'mirror' and not the 'sun'. They do not look for the rays of the soul beyond the 'mirror'. They judge the patient according to their own values and find the result disappointing. Care-givers are the co-travellers of patients with Alzheimer's disease, patients who need to complete their journey through this world with the help of their friends and loved ones.

This journey is too difficult for the patient to bear alone. The co-travellers, for their part, will discover new mysteries with respect to the reality of this journey of life. Although it is a very strenuous, physically difficult journey, it is also a spiritual companionship. It is an act of faith more than an act of reason.

The act of caring for an ill person should, however, be viewed not only as being beneficial to the recipient but also as being a positive experience for the giver. Not only our own suffering but also the suffering of our friends and loved ones challenges us to grow, through caring for them and sharing their sorrow and misery. The sickness of a relative or loved one gives us a chance to test to what degree our attributes of forbearance and patience have developed.

The following story demonstrates this principle:

> Lua Getsinger, one of the early Bahá'ís of America . . . had made the pilgrimage to the prison-city to see 'Abdu'l-Bahá. She was with Him one day when He said to her that He was too busy that day to call upon a friend of His who was very ill and poor. He wished Lua to go in His place.
>
> 'Take him food,' He said, 'and care for him as I have been doing.' He told her where this man was to be found, and she went gladly, proud that 'Abdu'l-Bahá should trust her to do some of His own work.
>
> Lua went, but she returned quickly. 'Master,' she exclaimed, 'surely you cannot realize to what a terrible place you sent me! I almost fainted from the awful smells, the dirty rooms, the low condition of that man and his house. I ran away before I should catch some terrible disease.'

'Abdu'l-Bahá looked at her sadly and like a firm father. 'If you want to serve God,' He said, 'you must serve your fellow man, for in him do you see the image and likeness of God.' He then told her to go back to the man's house. 'If the house is dirty,' He said, 'you should clean it; if this brother of yours is not clean, bathe him; if he is hungry, feed him. Do not return until this is done. Many times 'Abdu'l-Bahá has done this for him; cannot you serve him even once?"[28]

Misconceptions about Alzheimer Patients

There are a number of myths and misconceptions about patients with Alzheimer's disease, one of which is that because of the loss of memory these patients do not suffer much from the impact of the illness. But close observation indicates that unless the illness is in an advanced stage, many of these patients show an intuitive awareness and painful realization of their intellectual impairment, which they very often deny. Another misconception is that, through intellectual stimulation, the care-giver can help patients regain their lost memory. Patients with Alzheimer's disease will continue to lose memory and the ability to learn new intellectual skills unless a treatment is found. On the other hand, some care-givers have found ways of helping their loved ones to use those faculties which remain. A care-giver writes: 'Gradually, I came to think of memory as a lake from which we draw what we need as we need it . . . I came to understand my most important service to my mother: to replace that lake of memories with a river of relevant information . . .'[29]

Mace and Rabins in their book *The 36-Hour Day* extensively discuss issues pertaining to caring for patients with Alzheimer's disease. They urge care-givers to avoid confrontation or argumentation. Life should be made as easy and as simple as possible, without complicated messages and signals. In normal circumstances, decisions are made on the basis of facts; but in Alzheimer patients, memory fails to assimilate and present the facts, and hence decisions are often irrelevant to current situations.

Another misconception arises from the fact that patients with Alzheimer's disease generally look healthy prior to their terminal stage. Because of this healthy appearance, care-givers and friends are at times reluctant to recognize or accept the tragic impairment taking place within the patient. 'When a person loses a limb, or eyesight, or has a heart attack,' writes one care-giver, 'we know that, along with physical care, help will be needed to enable the patient to deal with the non-physical consequences of this disaster which has occurred. In the case of Alzheimer's disease, it is that part of the person, the brain . . . which is, itself, debilitated.' We expect sufferers to remember and perform as well intellectually and emotionally as they appear physically. Instead, we need to help the patient 'come to terms with the most devastating experience of all: consciousness that he is losing the use of his precious power, the power which seems to distinguish him from an animal, the power to think clearly.'[30]

The Responsibility of the Care-Givers

Caring for a patient suffering from Alzheimer's disease is a commitment which may last many years. Family members or friends who assume the role of care-givers face an emotionally taxing responsibility. Their task requires daily exposure to their patients' psychological, social and physical needs.

Care-givers need to develop a sense of detachment in order to deal effectively with the demented individual. As explained earlier, our attitude towards a sick person is closely related to our understanding of the true nature of the human being. If we believe that people have only a material being then our judgement of the patient is more likely to be influenced by material considerations. However, if our perception of human reality is that people also have a spiritual nature, our judgement of an Alzheimer's patient will reflect this. We will see in the person a soul on its own spiritual journey.

O'Quin and McGraw[31] discuss extensively those factors which may play an important role in the quality of the care given to demented patients. One of these factors is age. Older care-givers may be at a greater disadvantage in fulfilling their caring tasks because of the decline of their own mental faculties and reduced physical and financial capacity. On the other hand, younger care-givers may have additional challenges to face such as fulfilling personal responsibilities – marriage, education, children, job, etc. Moreover, they may be constantly reminded, by the dementia of the Alzheimer patient, of their own possible susceptibility to this illness. (It has been estimated that the possibility of developing Alzheimer's disease increases fourfold among family members of a person suffering from this illness.)[32]

One of the most serious emotional problems facing care-givers is depression. Factors which would contribute to the development of depression in the care-givers are feelings of isolation, alienation from others and lack of an adequate support system. Other factors are feelings of hopelessness, failure and guilt. Demented patients by the very nature of their illness will become increasingly dependent on the care-giver. This, in turn, adds to the care-giver's sense of obligation. Absence of a support system provided by family or friends will deepen a feeling of helplessness and despair in the care-giver. Therefore, caring should not be defined as the permanent role of one particular individual, but rather as a task to be shared by several, using all other community resources available.

Stress in Caring for Alzheimer Patients

Caring for an Alzheimer patient can be very stressful, especially if the care-giver is related to the patient. Related care-givers come to this task with their personal memories of the past and cherished hopes for a future that will never be. As one care-giver lamented, 'Why my parents? They worked so hard; they deserved a happy life together after all those years!'

Regarding the stress experienced when caring for patients with Alzheimer's disease, there are certain factors which will influence one's ability to cope.[33] One of these factors is unpredictability. The less predictable a situation is, the greater will be the level of arousal and anxiety. Another factor is uncertainty. In circumstances and conditions where there is great uncertainty, a high level of stress is likely to be produced. This is because the processes for coping are frozen as the care-giver becomes less certain of what the appropriate response to a particular situation should be, thus disarming him as he prepares to cope. As unpredictability and uncertainty characterize behavioural changes of demented patients, such as those afflicted with Alzheimer's, these patients are capable of generating a great deal of distress and discomfort in the care-giver. Coping with stress in such circumstances requires patience, certitude and stability on the part of the care-giver.

In some respects the uncertainty of family members of Alzheimer patients resembles the uncertainty of women whose husbands are reported missing in combat areas. Being uncertain as to whether their husbands are alive or dead, these women experience severe frustration. Likewise, the spouse of an Alzheimer patient suffers from an uncertain present and an unpredictable future of his or her loved one. Part of the uncertainty stems from the fact that the patient is psychologically absent but physically present. The unpredictability lies in never knowing the life expectancy of the patient and when the patient will have, for a precious moment, the ability to recall and remember or to hold a normal conversation. These are challenges in the life of the care-giver which he or she must face and for which adaptive solutions must be found. These challenges may lead to creative ways of coping despite all the frustrations. Such challenges also cause us to reflect on the wisdom of submission to a Greater Will.

Caring for Care-Givers

Researchers George and Gwyther reported in their survey of 500 care-givers of demented patients that 54% of the care-givers were spouses, 33% were children, 10% were other relatives and only 3% were those who were paid care-givers.[34] Care-givers receive little recognition or support for their never-ending hours of tedious responsibilities. They are the 'hidden victims'[35] of Alzheimer's disease to whom society has given little attention.

Caring for a demented patient is a type of giving for which there is no return. With some rare exceptions, there is little expression of gratitude or acknowledgement from patients to brighten the days of their care-givers, as the patient's attention span, judgement and ability to recognize the loving care of others are usually too limited or impaired to be able to appreciate the value of these services. One of those rare moments is described by this care-giver, who had given her mother a massage: 'Mother could no longer utter a sound or evoke a grateful gesture, yet in her eyes was an ocean of love and appreciation and acceptance.'

Family members and other care-givers often feel guilty, thinking that they do not give enough; they may attribute the patient's deterioration to their own failure to care for him properly. Because of their constant involvement in caring, care-givers isolate themselves from others and hence make themselves more vulnerable to burn-out and exhaustion. In responding to their patients' needs, they overlook or deny their own, which results in feelings of anger and resentment.

A care-giver's attitude to the patient can be greatly influenced by repressed and unresolved feelings of anger and hostility. These feelings should be dealt with through therapy or counselling in order to make the contact with the patient more effective.

Care-givers need a great deal of support and reassurance. The following words of Bahá'u'lláh illustrate the great importance of their task: 'Should anyone give you a choice between the opportunity to render a service to Me and a service to them [parents], choose ye to serve them, and let such a service be a path leading you to Me.'[36]

In many parts of the world today there are local Alzheimer Societies where family members and other care-givers can meet on a regular basis and share their own views and feelings. Through such periodic contact they realize that they are not alone in their predicament and can discover new ways of coping and caring for their loved ones. Care-givers not only need to be understood but they also need to be relieved periodically from their burden of caring so that they may attend to their own needs and regain their strength.

The Role of Society

Society plays an important role in the rehabilitation of Alzheimer patients and in helping care-givers to cope. It should provide both patients and their families with support systems which will enable the process of caring to continue. The feeling of helplessness and despair so commonly observed in family members and care-givers suggests that coping with patients is a very tedious task. Local Alzheimer Societies constitute an integral part of a support system for care-givers. However, because psychological, biological, environmental and spiritual needs of individuals vary, different ways of adapting to and coping with Alzheimer patients should be provided. The multitude of needs of Alzheimer patients requires a multidisciplinary and comprehensive approach. On the physical level, society should provide shelter and care facilities, e.g. nursing homes and similar institutions for patients. On the psychological level, it should provide counselling and support for the care-givers so that they can cope with the long-term effects of this chronic illness. It should educate care-givers on the nature and evolution of the illness and sensitize people in the community to the emotional needs of care-givers. (Our hospital systems concentrate primarily on the patient and not on the family.) In its environmental role, the community should provide a healing and supportive climate by creating a number of support networks and agencies with resources available to ailing patients.

In the spiritual realm, we must come to recognize the nobility of the individual behind the shadow of the illness. Prayers and meditation, as complementary therapy, are very uplifting to the soul. In the Bahá'í community, the Spiritual Assembly can provide spiritual guidance and understanding of the human journey. The following is a letter written by a Spiritual Assembly to an Alzheimer patient who was still able to understand and to receive advice which she was otherwise reluctant to accept from her family members and friends.

Dear . . .
Since becoming a Bahá'í you have been a constant, devoted

and loyal servant of Bahá'u'lláh. You can look back on many services to the Faith such as . . . the raising of a daughter who in turn is a loyal and devoted servant of Bahá'u'lláh. '*Rarely does it happen that a father and mother in this world see the reward of the care and trouble they have undergone for their children.*'[37]

You have lived to see it.

Through the natural process of ageing, you are now moving into a new stage of a long and useful life. Along with thousands of others in this country, you are now being subjected to Alzheimer's disease. The combined effects of this disease and physical ageing are considerable. Sometimes your memory works and other times it doesn't. Sometimes you lose track of what time of day it is or even what city you are in, and this can be embarrassing. It is important to realize, however, that you are not responsible for this decline in powers. As 'Abdu'l-Bahá says, 'nothing which exists remains in a state of repose – that is to say, all things are in motion. Everything is either growing or declining.'[38]

To a believer in a similar situation the Guardian wrote that such illnesses 'have nothing to do with our spirit or our inner relation to God'.[39] 'Abdu'l-Bahá says: '*The mind is circumscribed, the soul limitless. It is by the aid of such senses as those of sight, hearing, taste, smell and touch, that the mind comprehendeth, whereas, the soul is free from all agencies . . . the soul is ever endowed with full strength.*'[40]

It is when our physical powers fail that we can deeply understand the meaning of 'I testify, at this moment, to my powerlessness and to Thy might, to my poverty and to Thy wealth'.[41] Surely there is no stronger reminder of our powerlessness than a disease that deprives us, not only of our physical strength, but even our mental capacity. In fact this loss of powers can be the stimulus to a further stage of the soul's development – to see our true independence as reliance upon God. Unlike our physical powers which are not needed in the life to come, such spiritual growth is essential to our existence in the next world.

At this time of life you need some care, you can no longer

look after yourself alone. In the 'Words of Wisdom' Bahá'u'lláh says: *'The source of all glory is acceptance of whatsoever the Lord hath bestowed, and contentment with that which God hath ordained.'*[42]

If you can let go of your understanding of independence and accept that need for care, letting others be aware of your needs, you create an opportunity for others to serve. When you accept the need for care your fragility becomes a gift because it gives others that opportunity to care for you. Many of us . . . would welcome the opportunity to assist you. It's the best way we can show our love for you! In such a situation the Guardian wrote: *'. . . although in some ways you may be a . . . burden to your children, it is to them a privilege to look after you; you are their Mother and have given them life, and through the bounty of Bahá'u'lláh they are now attracted to His Faith. Anything they do for you is small recompense for all you have done for them.'*[43]

. . .We feel it is a privilege to have you in our community and are eager to show our love for you by assisting in any way we can with challenges now facing you.

With deepest love,
*Spiritual Assembly of
the Bahá'ís of . . .*

Some Suggestions for Caring

The following are some thoughts and suggestions with respect to caring for patients with Alzheimer's disease.

* We need to reassess our attitudes towards pain and suffering and to recognize the role of these difficulties in our personal growth and fulfilment. 'Abdu'l-Bahá explains that in this world we are influenced by two sentiments, joy and pain. He emphasizes that there is no human being who is not influenced by these two sentiments, 'but all the sorrow and the grief that exist come from the world of matter – the spiritual world bestows only joy! If we suffer

it is the outcome of material things, and all the trials and troubles come from this world of illusion.'[44] Caring for old and ageing people with or without dementia is a personal challenge that can give a new meaning to our lives. It helps us to grow spiritually and moves us away from our self-centredness. To show love and to care for someone who is helpless and impaired will help us to develop the virtues we need in our journey through this world. It will serve as an impetus for spiritual growth. A psychologist who specialized in studying the effect on personal growth of caring for a relative with Alzheimer's disease writes: 'The care-giving process provides . . . the spiritual dimension.'[45]

- We need to pray and meditate with the patient whenever possible. The creative words of the divine Manifestation are invested with a potency that can comfort the soul and alleviate pain and suffering as they unfold the meaning and mystery of life before us. It is not always possible for a demented person to pay full attention when a prayer is recited, but this does not mean that person's soul is unaware of the prayerful moment spent with others.

- We need to discover certain clues that make contact with these patients more practical and possible. Presenting objects which trigger memories, such as a favourite flower or a special piece of music, may have a therapeutic effect on the patient. Once I visited an Alzheimer patient in a nursing home. She could no longer articulate words clearly or remember things. I took her some fresh mint and lilac which she had always liked very much. The smell of the mint lit up her face and she sniffed it repeatedly; seeing her favourite flowers also evoked a special feeling.

I was told that she used to play the violin when she was very young. I suggested to the family that they bring recordings of her favourite violin pieces and play them for her, as this might evoke good feelings of the past. Can hearing a favourite piece of music or seeing a special flower or a family picture call up memories of these things in patients? Although I cannot say with certainty, the expression of patients I have seen leads me to believe that this is a possibility, if the illness is not too advanced. Perhaps a flashback of feeling rather than intellectual awareness can be evoked through these experiences.

In another case, a 78-year-old patient was reported to have been happy only at the birthday celebration of one of her grandchildren when she spontaneously started to sing 'Happy Birthday'. Those precious moments, a reminder of the past, were her only fleeting contact with the world of reality. After the birthday celebration she slipped back into her world of confusion. Similarly, prayers are like spiritual cues which evoke a feeling of inner assurance and delight.

'The loss of memory generates a forest of fears. Perhaps the most common one derives from having forgotten where you are,' writes one care-giver. Finding clues to help an Alzheimer's patient regain a sense of where they are is not easy, however. Elizabeth Rochester, a professional social worker with profound insight gained through the illness of her own mother, shows us how it can be done: 'Once I visited a woman in a nursing home who was in an advanced stage of Alzheimer's disease, her body rock-hard with tension, her face anxious, her manner angry. I remember her as a cheerful, welcoming hostess, interested in everyone and everything in the whole world.

'I noticed the repetition, "I don't know where my home is." Immediately I set to work to try to understand the real meaning of the question and to discover the needed 'real answer'. My first thought was that this woman no longer had a home. Then I remembered the book *Life After Life*.[46] Many who had had near-death experiences described a figure of light, or some relative, who came to meet them. This woman, a Bahá'í, had a picture by her bed of 'Abdu'l-Bahá, the son of the Founder of the Bahá'í Faith, for whom she felt great love and trust.

'When I was leaving I told this woman, a friend of forty years, that I wanted to say goodbye.

' "I don't know where my home is."

' "I know, and it's all right. 'Abdu'l-Bahá knows where you are and, when the time is right, He will come for you and take you home."

'She watched me intently and I had the sense that she understood.

'Six months later, after others had followed this example, my friend was more relaxed. Recently she had her teeth extracted and the gums sewn up; she was in misery; she turned to the picture and said, "It is time now. It is time for me to go into the picture." '[47]

Using past experiences to reorient a confused patient can also prove to be very helpful. The wife of an Alzheimer patient who had to be placed in a nursing home related the following incident to the author. 'One day my husband was so agitated that the nurses had to strap him to his bed or his wheelchair for his own safety. He protested about his "incarceration" and expressed his displeasure to me when I arrived. He wanted to know where he was, who these people were and he demanded to be taken home. I was able to calm him by telling him, "You see we are on a trip and we have travelled in the past quite a lot. Now we are on another journey and, for the time being, are staying at this place, but later on we will be going to a much more comfortable place. When we travelled by car, we used to buckle up for safety. Here, you need the strap for your safety because we are on a trip." He was comforted by this reassurance and accepted the situation.'

• We need to accept patients as they are, and not as they used to be or as they 'ought' to be. A relative of an Alzheimer's patient once commented, 'The worst is that he is not the same! He used to have such a good sense of humour and loved to dance. Now he just sits there in a corner and looks miserable all the time.'[48] Often, the family and friends of an Alzheimer's patient compare the patient as he is now to the way he used to be. This kind of judgemental comparison makes the task of caring and coping more tedious. Alzheimer's patients cannot be changed by our wishing them to do so, but we can make life easier for them. We must reflect and meditate on the nobility of a human being in creation and respect this nobility under all conditions of the journey through this world. Illness is a condition which we do not choose but which comes to us as a challenge.

• We need to be aware that the elderly, especially patients with Alzheimer's disease, are frightened of rejection and of being abandoned by their family members and friends. This view generates a great deal of anxiety and insecurity. They need to be frequently reassured, through verbal and physical expressions of love and affection, that they will not be abandoned.

• We should try to keep the patient at home for as long as possible, since it is an environment which is secure and familiar. The impersonal and sterile atmosphere of many professional institutions, where constant family contact is absent, can reinforce patients' belief that they are being abandoned.

Care at home, however, is not always possible. The onset of the terminal stage of the disease and the need for constant care, particularly medical care, may make it necessary to give consideration to nursing homes or similar environments. This separation can create a great deal of anguish and guilt in family members. In fact, on a questionnaire administered by the author, 'putting him (or her) into a home' was the most common response to the question, 'What was your most difficult or painful moment in caring for your loved one?' On the other hand, one care-giver looked upon her mother's move to a nursing home as 'pioneering' (settling in a new place as a Bahá'í to help spread the Faith in that area) and so did the mother! Dr Geila Bar-David in her research on the relatives of Alzheimer patients noted that children of Alzheimer patients tend to institutionalize their parents at an earlier stage of the illness than do spouses. This may be due to the fact that parents often live alone and need constant care. Moreover, children who have taken parents into their marital home have experienced many difficulties in trying to integrate them into their own family lives. However, spouses who are care-givers tend to prevent their children from assuming a large part of the responsibility of care-giving as they fear that this may burden their children who may have their own problems. It was also noted that daughters are more likely than sons to become the care-givers of the patient.[49]

- Regardless of whether we are able to keep the patient at
  home or feel that placing him in a nursing home is best,
  the Bahá'í Writings remind us that while we are still in
  this world, we should prepare our souls by acquiring
  divine virtues which are essential for the progress of our
  souls in the next world. 'Abdu'l-Bahá states: 'When our
  thoughts are filled with the bitterness of this world, let us
  turn our eyes to the sweetness of God's compassion and
  He will send us heavenly calm! If we are imprisoned in the
  material world, our spirit can soar into the heavens and we
  shall be free indeed! When our days are drawing to a close
  let us think of the eternal worlds, and we shall be full of
  joy!'[50]

Although devastating, Alzheimer's disease can provide
opportunities for spiritual growth. Memory loss, for example,
can be seen to convey a positive symbolic meaning – the
disappearance of the acquired knowledge of this world. The
mind becomes like a cup which empties the drops it has
gathered through the years and readies itself to be filled with
fresh water from the world of divine reality. As one care-giver
put it, 'I have meditated much on the spiritual value that such
an illness could possible have. One hint comes from the *Seven
Valleys* where Bahá'u'lláh says that the Valley of Knowledge is
the last plane of limitation. Maybe there are times when the
All-Merciful must physically remove this plane from us to give
our souls a chance to prepare for real flight.' The impact of
that flight is described by the daughter of an Alzheimer
victim: 'When my mother passed away it was as if a vial of her
pure essence was poured out on our entire family . . . It was
not just that she had been released from the prison of her
body, but through the long illness that had demanded such

tremendous patience and attention to what was really essential in life (love) she had really become an angel. The spiritual presence during those days after her death was light and joyful, and full of love . . .'

7

Ageing: A Spiritual Perspective

The process of ageing involves the fulfilment of human potential. It can be compared to the life cycle of a flower which germinates, grows, forms a bud, blossoms and, in its final stage of growth, unfolds into its full beauty. The flower, however, like all material beings, following the culmination of its physical maturity, withers and dies. The human being, on the other hand, possessing a soul and a spiritual destiny, does not suffer the same fate.

The Evolution of the Soul

This difference in the pattern of evolution has been explained in the following passage from 'Abdu'l-Bahá:

> Absolute repose does not exist in nature. All things either make progress or lose ground. Everything moves forward or backward, nothing is without motion. From his birth, a man progresses physically until he reaches maturity, then, having arrived at the prime of his life, he begins to decline, the strength and powers of his body decrease, and he gradually arrives at the hour of death. Likewise a plant progresses from the seed to maturity, then its life begins to lessen until it fades and dies. A bird soars to a certain height and having reached the highest possible point in its flight, begins its descent to earth.
>
> Thus it is evident that movement is essential to all existence. All material things progress to a certain point, then begin to

decline. This is the law which governs the whole physical creation.

Now let us consider the soul. We have seen that movement is essential to existence; nothing that has life is without motion. All creation, whether of the mineral, vegetable or animal kingdom, is compelled to obey the law of motion; it must either ascend or descend. But with the human soul, there is no decline. Its only movement is towards perfection; growth and progress alone constitute the motion of the soul . . .

'Progress' is the expression of spirit in the world of matter. The intelligence of man, his reasoning powers, his knowledge,

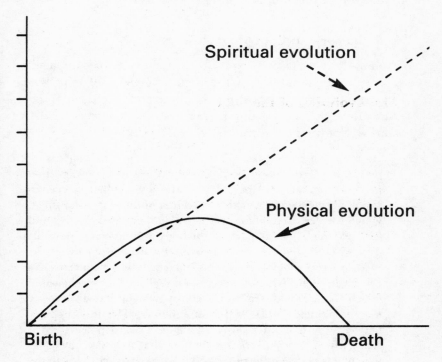

Physical and Spiritual Evolution of Human Beings

his scientific achievements, all these, being manifestations of the spirit, partake of the inevitable law of spiritual progress and are, therefore, of necessity, immortal.[1]

Therefore, the spiritual evolution of man does not follow the material pattern of ascent and decline. Whereas in the latter a period of growth is followed by decline and eventual death, in the former no such decline or death occurs. Although the extent of this progress varies from one individual to another, the soul maintains a continuous course of advancement. The diagram on the previous page illustrates the comparative evolution of the soul and the physical body.

The Sensory and Spiritual Powers

Although there are no specific Bahá'í Writings on ageing, there are explanations of the organic growth of man which enable us to have some understanding of our development. According to 'Abdu'l-Bahá, there are five physical and five spiritual powers operating in a human being:

> In man five outer powers exist, which are the agents of perception – that is to say, through these five powers man perceives material beings. These are sight, which perceives visible forms; hearing, which perceives audible sounds; smell, which perceives odours; taste, which perceives foods; and feeling, which is in all parts of the body and perceives tangible things. These five powers perceive outward existences.
>
> Man has also spiritual powers: imagination, which conceives things; thought, which reflects upon realities; comprehension, which comprehends realities; memory, which retains whatever man imagines, thinks and comprehends. The intermediary between the five outer powers and the inward powers is the sense which they possess in common, that is to say, the sense which acts between the outer and inner powers, conveys to the inward powers whatever the outer powers discern. It is termed

the common faculty, because it communicates between the
outward and inward powers and thus is common to the
outward and inward powers.

For instance, sight is one of the outer powers; it sees and
perceives this flower, and conveys this perception to the inner
power – the common faculty – which transmits this perception
to the power of imagination, which in its turn conceives and
forms this image and transmits it to the power of thought; the
power of thought reflects and, having grasped the reality,
conveys it to the power of comprehension; the comprehension,
when it has comprehended it, delivers the image of the object
perceived to the memory, and the memory keeps it in its
repository.[2]

In accordance with the patterns of evolution previously
described, the powers of the physical senses decline as one
ages. But the powers of the intellect do not follow a parallel
decline.

The Decline of the Physical Senses

As a person ages there is a decrease in sensitivity of all five
senses. The decline of vision is well-known. People over the
age of 65, for example, require almost 100 times as much
illumination as those in their twenties to see clearly a given
object in the presence of a glare.[3] Significant hearing loss is
estimated to occur in 2.8% of the population by the age of 55,
and by the age of 75, 15% are deaf.[4] Whereas a younger
person may be able to compensate for the weakness of one
sense by strengthening another, an elderly person's ability to
compensate will have greatly diminished.[5]

Intellectual Powers and Ageing

Turning to the intellectual powers, it has long been the

common belief that senility is the fate of every individual, given a long enough life span. However, some researchers now maintain that 'although the severe intellectual deterioration associated with senile dementia is often believed to be typical of old age, the diseases that cause dementia actually affect only a small proportion of the population'.[6] Estimates range between 5% and 7%.[7] Current research has shown that intellectual capacity remains stable until about the age of 67 and sometimes much later.[8]

One of the most widely held beliefs about ageing is that it is synonymous with memory loss. However, it has been shown that memory decline in a healthy elderly person is less extensive than was once thought. Although retrieval time may be longer, memory capacity seems to stay the same.[9] The most significant loss is in the ability to acquire new information. However, once something has been learned, an aged individual will remember it nearly as well as one who is younger.

Older persons often comment that they remember the more distant past more readily than recent events. Little research has been conducted on this subject because of the difficulty in determining which events are more or less recent. However, it can be argued that the past events that an elderly person remembers are usually major life events, such as a marriage or the birth of a child, which have greater significance than more recent mundane ones. Also, the elderly enjoy reminiscing about 'the good old days' and it is clear that the more one thinks about something, the better one remembers it.

Spiritual Development Knows No Age

In the world of spirit, ageing has no meaning. It is therefore possible that a child of ten years may surpass a person of 90 in

the acquisition of divine attributes and wisdom. The limitation of time is one of the characteristics of this mortal life. In
the realm of the spirit there is no age or time, 'just eternal
youth, and the enjoyment of eternal life'.[10] That is why there
is no age limit for those serving the Bahá'í Faith. It is a
spiritual affair and, unless one suffers from a physical
infirmity, age should not be seen as an impediment. Thus,
when the Guardian of the Bahá'í Faith was asked at what age
one should stop serving the Cause, he responded, 'There is no
age limit whatsoever for serving the Cause in administrative
capacities after one has reached twenty-one years. Indeed we
are supposed to serve the Cause to our last breath.'[11]

The spirit or soul is not only unaffected by age but also
untouched by diseases. Bahá'u'lláh wrote:

> That a sick person showeth signs of weakness is due to the
> hindrances that interpose themselves between his soul and his
> body, for the soul itself remaineth unaffected by any bodily
> ailments. Consider the light of the lamp. Though an external
> object may interfere with its radiance, the light itself continueth
> to shine with undiminished power. In like manner, every
> malady afflicting the body of man is an impediment that
> preventeth the soul from manifesting its inherent might and
> power. When it leaveth the body, however, it will evince such
> ascendancy, and reveal such influence as no force on earth can
> equal.[12]

Spiritual Health

Reassured by Bahá'u'lláh of the temporary nature of any ill
health that we may suffer in life, let us turn our attention to
the much neglected area of spiritual health. As compared to
physical health, this aspect of our existence is often ignored by
the medical profession. Yet spiritual health is of paramount

importance to the well-being of mankind. 'Abdu'l-Bahá
emphatically states,

> Pray that the spiritual health of mankind may be improved
> daily, for there are many doctors who attend to the physical
> ailments of the people, but there are very few divine
> physicians. It is in this connection that Christ said: 'Do not be
> afraid of those people who have control over your body, but
> have fear of those who may control your spirit.' Let your spirit
> be free so that it may soar toward the heights of sanctity. Let
> your spirit unfold the white wings of progress. Often physical
> sickness draws man nearer unto his Maker, suffers his heart to
> be made empty of all worldly desires until it becomes tender
> and sympathetic toward all sufferers and compassionate to all
> creatures. Although physical diseases cause man to suffer
> temporarily, yet they do not touch his spirit. Nay, rather, they
> contribute toward the divine purpose; that is, spiritual
> susceptibilities will be created in his heart.[13]

Preparation for the Next World

Life in this world can be compared to the nine months the
foetus spends in the womb of its mother. During this period of
confinement the yet-to-be-born individual is preparing for life
in this world. The perfection of the limbs and organs of an
unborn child is essential to enable that child to adjust and to
grow in this world. Similarly, human growth and the
fulfilment of one's spiritual potential in this world prepares
the soul for the world to come. The latter part of our life in this
world is, therefore, a final preparation for that stage. 'Abdu'l-
Bahá compares these two processes:

> In the beginning of his human life man was embryonic in the
> world of the matrix. There he received capacity and endow-
> ment for the reality of human existence. The forces and powers

necessary for this world were bestowed upon him in that limited condition. In this world he needed eyes; he received them potentially in the other. He needed ears; he obtained them there in readiness and preparation for his new existence. The powers requisite in this world were conferred upon him in the world of the matrix, so that when he entered this realm of real existence he not only possessed all necessary functions and powers but found provision for his material sustenance awaiting him.

Therefore in this world he must prepare himself for the life beyond. That which he needs in the world of the Kingdom must be obtained here. Just as he prepared himself in the world of the matrix by acquiring forces necessary in this sphere of existence, so likewise the indispensable forces of the divine existence must be potentially attained in this world.[14]

In preparation for the next world we need instruments which will enable us to progress and prosper there. These instruments are divine virtues and attributes which are to be acquired in the world of existence. Like the physical organs – limbs and senses developed during the embryonic world which enable us to function and maintain organic growth in this world – the divine attributes enable us to fulfil our potential in the world beyond.

Needs of the Next World

'What is [man] in need of in the Kingdom which transcends the life and limitation of this mortal sphere?' asked 'Abdu'l-Bahá. Then He Himself answered,

That world beyond is a world of sanctity and radiance; therefore it is necessary that in this world he should acquire these divine attributes. In that world there is need of spirituality, faith, assurance, the knowledge and love of God. These he must attain in this world so that after his ascension

from the earthly to the heavenly Kingdom he shall find all that
is needful in that life eternal ready for him.

The divine world is manifestly a world of lights; therefore
man has need of illumination here. That is a world of love; the
love of God is essential. It is a world of perfections; virtues or
perfections must be acquired. That world is vivified by the
breaths of the Holy Spirit; in this world we must seek them.
That is the Kingdom of life everlasting; it must be attained
during this vanishing existence.[15]

Having recognized our spiritual needs and identified the
instruments for their realization, we must discover the means
to acquire heavenly attributes. Once again, 'Abdu'l-Bahá
comes to our aid, listing seven ways to acquire spiritual
qualities.

First, through the knowledge of God.

Second, through the love of God.

Third, through faith.

Fourth, through philanthropic deeds.

Fifth, through self-sacrifice.

Sixth, through severance from this world.

Seventh, through sanctity and holiness.

He then warns, 'Unless [man] acquires these forces and
attains to these requirements he will surely be deprived of the
life that is eternal.'[16]

The Rewards of Life in this World and the Next

As we grow old we often wonder about the mysteries and
rewards of this life and what lies ahead for us in the world to
come. The Bahá'í Faith provides a clue. 'Abdu'l-Bahá states:

The rewards of this life are the virtues and perfections which adorn the reality of man . . . Through these rewards he gains spiritual birth and becomes a new creature . . . The rewards of the other world are the eternal life which is clearly mentioned in all the Holy Books, the divine perfections, the eternal bounties and everlasting felicity . . . peace, the spiritual graces, the various spiritual gifts in the Kingdom of God, the gaining of the desires of the heart and the soul, and the meeting of God in the world of eternity.[17]

References

Introduction

1. McPherson, Barry D., *Aging as a Social Process – An Introduction to Individual and Population Aging* (Toronto: Butterworths, 1983), p. 45
2. ibid.
3. ibid. p. 59.
4. ibid.
5. Timiras, Paola S., *Psychological Basis of Geriatrics* (New York: Macmillan Publishing Co., 1988), p. 4.
6. Bruner, Marcia, 'Aging', *A Doctor's Review* (March 1990), p. 156.
7. McPherson, *Aging as a Social Process*, pp. 6–10.
8. Zarit, Judy M. and Zarit, Steven H. 'Molar Aging: The Physiology and Psychology of Normal Aging', in Carstensen, Laura L., and Edelstein, Barry A., (eds), *Handbook of Clinical Gerontology* (New York: Pergamon Press, 1987), p. 22.
9. ibid.
10. ibid.
11. ibid.
12. ibid.
13. Vaillant, George E. and Vaillant, Caroline O., 'Natural History of Male Psychosocial Health, XII: A 45-Year Study of Predictors of Successful Aging at Age 65'. *American Journal of Psychiatry*, vol. 147, no. 1, January 1990, p. 31.
14. ibid. p. 34.
15. ibid. p. 36.
16. ibid.
17. Oldham, John M. and Liebart, Robert S. *The Middle Years: New*

Psychoanalytical Perspectives (New Haven, Ct.: Yale University Press, 1989).
18. Erikson, Erik, *Childhood and Society* (New York: W.W. Norton and Co., Inc., 1963), pp. 247–69.
19. Vaillant and Vaillant, 'Natural History', p. 31.

1. Our Ageing Society: Some Statistics and Reflections

1. Levinson, Daniel J. *The Seasons of a Man's Life* (New York: Ballentine Books, 1978), pp. 209–10.
2. ibid.
3. Ogden Nash, cited in Butler, R.N., and Bearne, A.G. (eds), *The Aging Process: Therapeutic Implications* (New York: Raven Press, 1985), p. 2.
4. Butler, 'A Changing Demography', in ibid. p. 6.
5. Dychtwald, *Wellness and Health Promotion for the Elderly* (Rockeville, Maryland: Aspen Publishers, 1986), p. 1.
6. ibid. p. 2.
7. United Nations, *Vienna International Plan of Action on Aging* (New York: United Nations, 1983), p. 14.
8. Butler, Robert N. 'Geriatric Psychiatry', in Kaplan, H.I., and Sadock, B.J., *Comprehensive Textbook of Psychiatry* (Baltimore: Williams and Wilkins, 1985), p. 1953.
9. ibid.
10. Dychtwald, *Wellness and Fitness*, pp. 1–17.
11. Butler, 'Geriatric Psychology', p. 1953.
12. ibid. p. 1954.
13. Dychtwald, *Wellness and Health*, p. 1.
14. United States Senate Special Committee on Aging and American Association of Retired Persons, *Aging America: Trends and Proportions*, 1984.
15. Rosenwike, I., Yaffe, N., and Sagi, P. 'The Recent Decline in Mortality of the Extreme Aged: An Analysis of Statistical Data', in *American Journal of Public Health*, 1980, no. 70, pp. 1074–90.
16. Butler, 'Changing Demography', pp. 5–6.
17. Dychtwald, *Wellness and Health*, p. 12.
18. Bruner, 'Aging', in *Doctor's Review*, March 1990, p. 155.
19. Dychtwald, *Wellness and Health*, p. 12.
20. *Journal of Current Therapy*, February 1989, vol. 2, no. 1, p. 30.

21. Dychtwald, *Wellness and Health*, p. 21.
22. ibid.
23. Henig, Robin Marantz, *The Myth of Senility* (Garden City, New York: Anchor Press – Doubleday, 1981), p. 13.

2. The Psychobiological Clock

1. Moore-Ede, Martin C., Sulzman, Frank M., and Fuller, Charles A. *The Clocks That Time Us* (Cambridge, Mass.: Harvard University Press, 1982), pp. 1–3.
2. Ghadirian, A-M., 'Human Responses to Life Stress and Suffering', *Bahá'í Studies Notebook: The Divine Institution of Marriage*. March 1983, vol. 3, nos. 1 and 2, pp. 49–62.
3. Bibring, Grete L. 'Old Age: Its Liabilities and Assets – A Psychological Discourse', in Loewenstein, Rudolph M., Newman, Lottie M., Schur, Max, and Solnut, Albert J. (eds), *Psychoanalysis – A General Psychology* (New York: International University Press, 1966), p. 257.
4. ibid. p. 268.
5. ibid. p. 265.
6. ibid. p. 262.
7. ibid.
8. Lieberman, Morton A. and Tobin, Sheldon S. *The Experience of Old Age – Stress, Coping and Survival* (New York: Basic Books, 1983), p. 3.
9. Bahá'u'lláh, *The Hidden Words of Bahá'u'lláh* (Wilmette, Illinois: Bahá'í Publishing Trust, 1985), Arabic, no. 11.

3. Ageing and Creativity

1. 'Abdu'l-Bahá, *The Promulgation of Universal Peace* (Wilmette, Illinois: Bahá'í Publishing Trust, 1982), p. 438.
2. Tuli, Jitendra, 'Where Age Brings Honor', in *World Health Magazine*, February–March, 1982, p. 23.
3. Mahler, Halfden, 'Add Life to Years', in *World Health Magazine*, February–March, 1982, p. 3.
4. Pruyser, Paul, 'Creativity in Aging Persons', in *Bulletin of the Menninger Clinic*, 1987, vol. 51, no. 5, p. 425–35.
5. Mahler, 'Add Life to Years', p. 3.

6. Dychtwald, *Wellness and Health*, p. 13.
7. *Encyclopedia Britannica*, 1988, vol. 24, p. 868.
8. 'They Defied Old Age . . .', in *World Health Magazine*, February–March 1982, pp. 36–7.
9. *Encyclopedia Britannica*, 1988, vol. 25, p. 868.
10. 'They Defied Old Age . . .', p. 36.
11. Abu'l-Faḍl Gulpáygání, Mírzá, *Miracles and Metaphors* (Los Angeles, Calif.: Kalimát Press, 1981), pp. xviii, xiv.
12. *Encyclopedia Britannica*, 1988, vol. 28, pp. 708–9.
13. Stendardo, Luigi, *Leo Tolstoy and the Bahá'í Faith* (Oxford: George Ronald, 1985).
14. Fischer, Louis, *Gandhi, His Life and Message for the World* (New York: Mentor Books, 1954), p. 154.
15. *The Bahá'í World* (Wilmette, Illinois: Bahá'í Publishing Committee, 1945), 1940–1944, vol. IX, p. 613.
16. *The Bahá'í World* (Wilmette, Illinois: Bahá'í Publishing Trust, 1949), 1944–1946, vol. X, p. 519.
17. Kramer, Rita, *Maria Montessori* (New York: G.P. Putnam's Sons, 1976), pp. 349–67.
18. Lash, Joseph P., *Eleanor: The Years Alone* (New York: W.W. Norton and Co., 1972), pp. 302–3, 331.
19. Freud, Sigmund, *On Psychotherapy* (London: Hogart Press, 1953), Standard Edition, vol. 7, p. 257.
20. Wasylenki, Donald A. 'Psychodynamics and Aging', in *Canadian Journal of Psychiatry*, February 1982, vol. 27, p. 11.
21. French, A.P. (ed), *Einstein – A Centenary Volume* (Cambridge, Mass.: Harvard University Press, 1979), p. 32.
22. Cousins, Norman, *Anatomy of an Illness* (Toronto: Bantam Books, 1979), pp. 72–4.
23. ibid. pp. 79–82.
24. ibid. p. 85.
25. ibid. p. 86.
26. ibid.
27. Timiras, *Physiological Basis of Geriatrics*, p. 24.
28. ibid. pp. 24–5.
29. Butler, 'Changing Demography', pp. 7–8.
30. Hallowell, Christopher, *Growing Old, Staying Young* (New York: William Morrow and Co., 1985), p. 243.

4. The Challenges of Old Age

1. Dobbie, Judy, 'Substance Abuse among the Elderly', in *Addictions*, Fall 1977, pp. 1–2.
2. Bibring, Grete L. 'Old Age: Its Liabilities and Assets – A Psychological Discourse', in Loewenstein, Rudolph M., Newman, Lottie M., Schur, Max and Solnut, Albert J., (eds), *Psychoanalysis – A General Psychology* (New York: International University Press, 1966), p. 264.
3. 'Families Provide Bulk of Care to Persons with Alzheimer's Disease and Other Dementias', in *Hospital and Community Psychiatry*, September 1987, vol. 38, no. 9, p. 1004.
4. Jacques, Alan, *Understanding Dementia* (Edinburgh: Churchill Livingstone, 1988), pp. 5–6.
5. 'Older – But Coming on Strong', in *Time Magazine*, 22 February 1988, p. 49.
6. Dobbie, 'Substance Abuse', p. 12.
7. ibid. p. 13.
8. ibid. p. 17.
9. Butler, 'Geriatric Psychiatry', p. 1955.
10. Ghadirian, A-M., 'Human Responses to Life Stress and Suffering', in *Association of Bahá'í Studies*, 1983, vol. 3, nos. 1 and 2, pp. 46–62.
11. Frankl, Viktor E., *Man's Search for Meaning: An Introduction to Logotherapy* (New York: Pocket Books, 1963), p. 179.
12. Sadock, Virginia A. 'Other conditions not attributable to a mental disorder' in Kaplan, Harold I., and Sadock, Benjamin J. (eds), *Comprehensive Textbook of Psychiatry*. (Baltimore: Williams and Wilkins, 4th ed., 1985), vol. 2, pp. 1872–7.
13. ibid.
14. ibid.
15. Butler, 'Geriatric Psychology', p. 1955.
16. Ghadirian, A-M., *In Search of Nirvana: A New Perspective on Alcohol and Drug Dependency* (Oxford: George Ronald, 2nd ed. 1989).
17. Hallowell, *Growing Old*, pp. 186–7.
18. ibid. pp. 181–200.
19. Plato, 'Trial and Death of Socrates', in Kuykendall, E., (ed), *Philosophy in the Age of Crisis*. (New York: Harper and Row, 1970), p. 14.

20. Kubler-Ross, Elisabeth, *On Death and Dying* (New York: Macmillan, 1969), pp. 38–137.
21. 'Abdu'l-Bahá in *Bahá'í World Faith* (Wilmette, Illinois: Bahá'í Publishing Trust, 1976), p. 379.
22. Bahá'u'lláh, *Hidden Words*, Arabic, no. 32.

5. Coping with Stress

1. Caplan, 'Master of Stress: Psychological Aspects', in *American Journal of Psychiatry*, 1981, vol. 138, no. 5, p. 414.
2. Patrick, P.K.S., 'Burnout: Job Hazard for Health Workers', in *J. Hospitals*, 16 November 1979, p. 87.
3. Selye, Hans, *Stress without Distress* (Scarborough, Ontario: A New American Library of Canada, 1974), p. 83.
4. Rees, W. Linford, 'Stress, Distress and Disease', in *British Journal of Psychiatry*, 1976, vol. 128, pp. 3–4.
5. Faizi, Gloria, *Stories About 'Abdu'l-Bahá* (New Delhi: Bahá'í Publishing Trust, 1981), pp. 11–12.
6. Pines, A.M., Aronson, E., and Kafry, D. 'Postscript: Burnout and Tedium Outside of Work', in Pines, Aronson and Kafry, *Burnout – from Tedium to Personal Growth* (New York: The Free Press, 1981), p. 172.
7. Fettes, I., 'Migraine Linked to Low Endorphins', quoted by Austin Rand in *Medical Post*, 26 July 1983, vol. 19, no. 15, p. 38.
8. 'Stress: Can We Cope?' *Time*, 6 June 1983, p. 57.
9. 'Abdu'l-Bahá, *The Divine Art of Living* (Wilmette, Illinois: Bahá'í Publishing Trust, rev. edn. 1960), p. 92.
10. ibid. p. 91.
11. 'Stress on the Job', *Newsweek*, 25 April 1988, p. 43.
12. Connidis, Ingrid, 'Life in Older Age: The View from the Top', in Marshall, V.W. (ed), *Aging in Canada – Social Perspectives* (Markham, Ontario: Fitzhenry and Whiteside, 1987), p. 469.
13. Bahá'u'lláh, *The Book of Certitude* (Wilmette, Illinois: Bahá'í Publishing Trust, 1950), p. 238.
14. 'Abdu'l-Bahá in *Bahá'í World Faith*, p. 363.
15. Cousins, *Anatomy of an Illness*, p. 44.
16. 'The A. A. Grapevine, Inc.', *Alcoholics Anonymous* (New York: A.A. World Service).

17. Bahá'u'lláh, *Gleanings from the Writings of Bahá'u'lláh* (Wilmette, Illinois: Bahá'í Publishing Trust, rev. edn. 1952), pp. 242–3.
18. McGrath, J.E., 'A Conceptual Formulation for Research on Stress', in McGrath, J.E. (ed), *Social and Psychological Factors in Stress* (New York: Holt, Rinehart and Winston, 1970), p. 18.
19. 'Stress: Can We Cope?' *Time*, 6 June 1983, p. 56.
20. 'Abdu'l-Bahá in *Star of the West*, vol. 12, no. 16, p. 250 (Oxford: George Ronald, reprinted 1978, vol. 7).
21. Sears, William, *God Loves Laughter* (Oxford: George Ronald, 1960).
22. Cousins, *Anatomy of an Illness*, pp. 39–40.
23. Honnold, Annamarie (ed), *Vignettes from the Life of 'Abdu'l-Bahá* (Oxford: George Ronald, 1982), pp. 150–1.
24. ibid. p. 151.
25. *Living the Life* (London: Bahá'í Publishing Trust, 1974), p. 18.
26. 'Abdu'l-Bahá in *The Reality of Man* (Wilmette, Illinois: Bahá'í Publishing Trust, 1962), pp. 15–16.
27. *The Unfolding Destiny of the British Bahá'í Community* (Oakham: Bahá'í Publishing Trust, 1981), pp. 456–7.

6. Alzheimer's Disease: An Eclipse Before Sunset

1. 'Abdu'l-Bahá, 'Tablet to Dr Forel', in *The Bahá'í Revelation* (London: Bahá'í Publishing Trust, 1955), p. 221.
2. Aronson, Miriam K., 'Alzheimer's and Other Dementias: A Major Public Health Problem', *Carrier Foundation Letter*, November 1981, p. 1.
3. *Diagnostic and Statistical Manual of Mental Disorders* (Washington DC: American Psychiatric Association, 3rd edn. 1987), p. 107.
4. Small, Gary W., 'Psychopharmocological Treatment of Elderly Demented Patients', *Journal of Clinical Psychiatry*, May 1988, vol. 49, no. 5 (Supplement), p. 8.
5. Glenner, George G. 'Alzheimer's Disease: The Pathology, the Patient, and the Family', in Hutton, Thomas J., and Kenny, Alexander D., (eds), *Senile Dementia of the Alzheimer Type* (New York: Alan R. Liss, 1985), p. 275.
6. ibid.
7. Personal communication from Elizabeth Rochester.
8. ibid.

9. 'Abdu'l-Bahá, *Some Answered Questions* (Wilmette, Illinois: Bahá'í Publishing Trust, rev. edn. 1981), p. 200.
10. 'Abdu'l-Bahá in *Bahá'í World Faith*, pp. 346–7.
11. Bahá'u'lláh, *Gleanings*, p. 155.
12. 'Abdu'l-Bahá, *Paris Talks* (London: Bahá'í Publishing Trust, 1969), p. 65.
13. Bahá'u'lláh, *Gleanings*, pp. 153–4.
14. 'Abdu'l-Bahá in *Reality of Man*, p. 9.
15. ibid. p. 10.
16. ibid. pp. 12–13.
17. Vader, John Paul, *For the Good of Mankind: August Forel and the Bahá'í Faith* (Oxford: George Ronald, 1984), p. 71.
18. Hornby, Helen (comp.), *Lights of Guidance: a Bahá'í Reference File* (New Delhi: Bahá'í Publishing Trust, rev. edn. 1988), p. 281, no. 948.
19. ibid.
20. Bahá'u'lláh in *Bahá'í Prayers* (Wilmette, Illinois: Bahá'í Publishing Trust, 1985), p. 90.
21. Zarit, Steven H., Orr, Nancy K., and Zarit, Judy M., *The Hidden Victims of Alzheimer's Disease – Families Under Stress* (New York: New York University Press, 1985), p. 96. By permission of the publisher.
22. ibid. p. 94.
23. ibid. p. 107.
24. 'Families Provide Bulk of Care', p. 1003.
25. Personal communication from Elizabeth Rochester.
26. ibid.
27. ibid.
28. Faizi, *Stories about 'Abdu'l-Bahá*, p. 3.
29. Personal communication from Elizabeth Rochester.
30. ibid.
31. O'Quin, Jo Ann, and McGraw, Kenneth O., 'The Burdened Caregiver: An Overview', in *Senile Dementia of the Alzheimer Type*, p. 68.
32. APA Joint Commission on Public Affairs and the Division of Public Affairs, 'Let's Talk Facts About: Mental Health in the Elderly' (Washington DC: American Psychiatric Association, 1988), p. 5.
33. Lazarus, Richard S., and Folkman, Susan, *Stress, Appraisal and*

Coping (New York: Springer Publishing Company, 1984), pp. 90–2.

34. O'Quin, Jo Ann, and McGraw, Kenneth O., 'The Burdened Caregiver', p. 68.
35. Zarit, Steven H., Orr, Nancy K., and Zarit, Judy M., *The Hidden Victims*, p. 94.
36. Bahá'u'lláh, cited in Hornby, *Lights of Guidance*, p. 530.
37. 'Abdu'l-Bahá, *Some Answered Questions*, p. 231.
38. ibid. p. 233.
39. Shoghi Effendi, cited in *Lights of Guidance*, p. 255.
40. 'Abdu'l-Bahá, in *Bahá'í World Faith*, pp. 337–8.
41. Bahá'u'lláh, in *Bahá'í Prayers*, p. 4.
42. Bahá'u'lláh, in *The Reality of Man* (Wilmette, Illinois: Bahá'í Publishing Trust, 1966), p. 3.
43. Shoghi Effendi, cited in *Lights of Guidance*, p. 230.
44. 'Abdu'l-Bahá, in *Reality of Man*, pp. 15–16.
45. Bar-David, Geila, 'Growing While Caring for a Relative with Alzheimer's Disease', a proposal for a Ph.D. thesis (unpublished).
46. Moody, Raymond A., *Life After Life* (New York: Bantam Books, 1975).
47. Personal communication from Elizabeth Rochester.
48. Bar-David, Geila, 'Growing While Caring for a Relative'.
49. ibid.
50. Abdu'l-Bahá, in *Reality of Man*, p. 16.

7. Ageing: A Spiritual Perspective

1. 'Abdu'l-Bahá in *Reality of Man*, pp. 18–19.
2. 'Abdu'l-Bahá, *Selections from the Writings of 'Abdu'l-Bahá* (Haifa: Bahá'í World Centre, 1978), pp. 210–11.
3. Fozard, J.L., and Popkins, S.J., 'Optimizing Adult Development: Ends and Means of an Applied Psychology of Aging', *American Psychologist*, 1978, vol. 33, pp. 975–89.
4. Zarit, Judy M., and Zarit, Steven, 'Molar Aging', p. 26.
5. ibid. p. 25.
6. ibid.
7. Mortimer, J.A., Schuman, L.M., and French, L.R., 'Epidemiology of Dementing Illness', in Mortimer, J.A., and Schuman, L.M., (eds), *The Epidemiology of Dementia* (New York: Oxford University Press, 1981), pp. 2–23.

8. Zarit, Judy M, and Zarit, Steven, 'Molar Aging', p. 30.
9. ibid. p. 28.
10. Letter of Shoghi Effendi to an individual believer, 19 May 1956, cited in a letter of the Universal House of Justice to an individual believer.
11. Letter of Shoghi Effendi to the National Spiritual Assembly of the Bahá'ís of India, 21 June 1953.
12. Bahá'u'lláh, *Gleanings*, p. 154.
13. Zohoori, Elias, (ed), *The Throne of the Inner Temple* (Jamaica: Elias Zohoori, 1985), pp. 20–1.
14. 'Abdu'l-Bahá, *Foundations of World Unity* (Wilmette, Illinois: Bahá'í Publishing Trust, 1945), p. 63.
15. ibid. pp. 63–4.
16. ibid. p. 64.
17. 'Abdu'l-Bahá, *Some Answered Questions*, pp. 223–5.

In Search of Nirvana

A New Perspective on Alcohol and Drug Dependency

by A-M. Ghadirian

Now in a new, completely revised, softcover edition

Dr Ghadirian's first book, *In Search of Nirvana*, reviews the medical research into the problems of alcohol and drug dependency and asks the question, 'What are the factors tending to lead to the abuse of these substances?'

Dr Ghadirian shows how the Bahá'í Faith uses a systematic and realistic approach to preventing substance abuse by focusing on early education, family life and the true nature of the individual. He draws together those Bahá'í principles which are concerned with the life of society and the community and demonstrates how, by applying these principles, the underlying factors leading to substance addition and abuse can be avoided.

'. . . merits serious attention by all concerned with this important social problem.' *Gerald L. Klerman, M.D., Professor of Psychiatry, Harvard Medical School.*

136 pages, softcover only
£4.50, US$8.95, Can$9.95　　　　　ISBN 0–85398–209–0

Bahá'í Families

Perspectives, Principles, Practice

by Patricia Wilcox

Here is a practical and down-to-earth guide to making your family a fortress for well-being.

Essential reading for families of all kinds, Patricia Wilcox draws on her own experience as a mother of five and a family counsellor to examine:

* the place of the family in world order
* unity in diversity within the family
* family consultation as a tool for progress
* the education of children

and the concept of divine education.

Available May 1992   **ISBN 0–85398–331–3**

Divine Therapy

Pearls of Wisdom from the Bahá'í Writings

compiled by Annamarie Honnold

This collection of quotations from the Bahá'í Sacred Writings offers vital help for emotional and spiritual healing.

Grouped in three sections, 'Coping with Stress', 'Orientation to the Divine' and 'Developing Helpful Attitudes', these 'pearls of wisdom' from the extensive literature of the Bahá'í Faith concentrate on common problems and their solution and are dedicated to 'all who seek inner peace and joy'.

224 pages, softcover only
£4.95, US$9.95, Can$10.95   ISBN 0–85398–237–6